MEDICAL MIRACLES

MY EXPERIENCES WITH LIFE

DR. PRADNYA .P. WALI

Dr. Pradnya P. Wali
1st Edition

Publication Date: April 2024
Price: ₹349 | $ 15
ISBN: 978-93-5847-230-1
Published by:
Adhyyan Books
Office No. 125,
Opposite Vivanta by Taj,
DDA SFS. Pocket-1, Dwarka,
Sec-22, New Delhi-110077
Website: http://adhyyanbooks.com
E-mail: contact@adhyyanbooks.com

Printed at: Repro Printers, Delhi

THIS WORK IS DEDICATED TO MY BELOVED GRANDMOTHER

LATE SMT AKKATAI KARAMBALI

AND

TO MY DEAR BROTHER

LATE DR VINAY.P.WALI

FOR HELPING US TO BE THE BEST VERSION OF OURSELVES AND FOR BEING A DIVINE GUIDANCE THROUGHOUT THE MEANDERING PATHS OF OUR LIVES.

PREFACE

Medical Miracles is a compilation of stories inspired by my real life clinical experiences of many years but presented in a fictional way. These are the stories of small kids suffering from various rare conditions but who overpowered their illnesses with great courage, strong willpower and never give up attitude. This book also presents the strong, determinative parents who went overboard to give better lives to their ailing children. My aim to write this book is to give scientific knowledge about various pediatric diseases in a very simple language which will be helpful and useful to every common man. The stories are kept simple and colloquial language has been retained in many stories to make it more real. The Hyderabadi Urdu mix Hindi is the soul of the story Hyderabadi Patient Nawaji and hence all the conversations have been kept in Hyderabadi slang to keep the naturality intact and I'm sure every die hard hyderabadi will relate to this story completely. The visible Gods and Human pyramid shows my respect to the Doctors who are serving the poor and needy selflessly for many decades now and are the torch bearers of this noble profession.

I salute from the bottom of my heart to all the brave fighters - my little patients, their ever supportive parents with great valor and all the Doctors who work hard relentlessly day and night to save every life. These stories bring rainbow of emotions and I have lived hundreds of lives in one with each and every character here. This book gives hope, positivity and encouragement to lead a happy life despite many life challenges and that's what makes it more special. These earthy characters of my stories are truly inspirational.

DR PRADNYA. P. WALI

ACKNOWLEDGEMENT

"When you really want something to happen, the whole universe conspires so that your wish comes true."

And yes with GOD's choicest blessings "**MEDICAL MIRACLES**" has truly happened today. In this journey, right from the beginning of making of medical miracles to final print and distribution of this book many people have helped and touched my life. And this book will be incomplete without extending my heartfelt gratitude towards their love and affection showered on me.

First and foremost I would like to thank the **ALMIGHTY GOD** for His never ending grace and provision during this entire process which ended up being one of my dreams come true moment.

My heartfelt gratitude for my Granny, Late **SMT AKKATAI KARAMBALI**, who has been a constant source of inspiration and driving force behind making of this book. Her words of wisdom, her strong willpower to tackles life's every odd has given me the vision to write these stories and to compile it in a book.

I would like to acknowledge the extraordinary debt I owe to

my parents, **DR PRAKASH WALI AND MRS KSHAMA WALI**, for their unwavering lifetime support and strong belief in me. My father has always been my Mentor, guide and best critic who always helped me to excel in all spheres of my life. Everything good in my life exists because of love, care and constant encouragement from my parents.

My heartfelt gratitude to my brother, Late **DR VINAY WALI**, for giving me wings to fly high and the courage to conquer this world. You were epitome of kindness, compassion and generosity who touched the hearts of poor and needy and filled their life with unending joys. Amidst a world full of chaos your selfless and ever helping nature has always inspired to be kind and my writing skills is indeed a genetic flow from you to me.

My deepest gratitude for my beloved sister **DR KSHITIJA WALI**, for her constant motivation and perseverance. She has been my biggest support system throughout my life. Without her unfailing and generous assistance and constructive ideas this project would not have been possible.

And to my lovely nephew **SRIVANSHU,** Thank you so much for adding colors and laughter in my life. Your full of life, cheerful attitude and radiating energy always encouraged me to continue my work tirelessly even after my mundane busy days.

I am grateful from bottom of my heart to my dear friend **Dr ASWAD KHAN**, for his understanding nature, patience, perseverance and for showing high level of tolerance in the most stressful times. Sharing his valuable inputs he also shared major responsibility at work front so that I could cater time for my writings. Our synergistic collaboration fostered a productive and positive work environment leading to completion of this project on time.

My heartfelt gratitude for my tiny warriors, **MY PATIENTS**, who imparted me with great knowledge and helped me sharpen my skills. Their unshaken strong willpower and fighting spirit inspired me to pen down these stories. You all are the **REAL HEROES** of my stories.

And then to the makers of **MEDICAL MIRACLES**, **ADDHYAN PUBLISHERS** and their entire **TEAM** for your valuable guidance, expert inputs and amazing skills to shape this Masterpiece.

I feel extremely privileged to be surrounded with such amazing people who made my life easy and helped me to tick one more wish from my **BUCKET LIST** successfully.

But I know this is just the beginning and I have many more things to accomplish miles to go before I sleep and miles to go before I sleep.

DR. PRADNYA.P.WALI

MAKING OF MEDICAL MIRACLES....

It was May 2020 when all of a sudden Nature went on a strike and our lives came to a complete halt. There was this bolt from the blue as COVID was on rise. It was almost 2 months now we all were in the lockdown. None of us ever thought that we will be caged animals and prisoners in our own houses. Sitting at my favourite French window one night after a heavy day and pondering at the serene sky thousands of twinkles filled my eye. A year ago i was in Thialand, jumping like jacks in that green safari and swimming deep in the blue sea like a thirsty whale. This time we had plan for the Swiss Alps and my mind was already wandering in those sky high mountains and my soul was shivering in those shimmery silvery ice-clad valleys. This very thought was indeed breath taking!

But COVID came and without a second thought our lives went for a total toss.The hustly bustly streets were suddenly barren. The malls, the Multiplexes, restaurants, Hifi-gyms, branded showrooms everything was shut without our notice. Only Locals were vocal. Small vendors were running their small shops and the little things we bought from these little shops showed us how little our basic needs were. Yes still we all lived and moreover we all survived! Nature laughed at us saying "Oh Man look, you too can survive with these tiny things. You just need what I created for you, the fresh air to breath, fresh food to eat and clean water to drink, above that what you have created for yourself is just too delicate to wither with time".

All these times we were busy running after earning livelihood forgetting our personal ties. In pride of building concrete jungles and the tallest buildings we encroached the nature's space, destroyed the wildlife habitats, Spoiled Sea water and flattened the tall beautiful mountains. We forgot sharing of feelings and caring for others. We were hungry for virtual fame, virtual looks and the virtual claps. Our real life was lost in the Virtual admiration!

And then one day Nature took strings in its hands and the Time machine was frozen! It showed us however smart and brainy we may be, we are nothing in front of it. It created just a 0.1 micronvirus to destroy the Supreme power of this world. Powerful Nations collapsed like a card castle in the air...! So I said Nature laughed at us showing how miniscule we were in front of it.

Being a Doctor and moreover an intensivist working in the highly sensitive zone of Neonatal ICU, I was juggling between my personal and professional life in this pandemic period. Maids disappeared and my life took a complete U turn. I was chopping veggies at one end while hearing to the update of the overnight ICU event on a phone call by my fellow colleague at NICU.I was counting whistles of cooker while calculating the fluid of a severely dehydrated baby. The time I was planning what to make for the breakfast my brain was mapping the oxygenation index of a baby on ventilator....!!

At work I was managing sick and critical babies but as the clock ticked 5 past half my brain was revising the list of "to do" things at my home. Buy vegetables, buy groceries, fill the petrol tank of my vehicle so that it continues it's marathon running without a stop.

True the Covid time was too hard and difficult but this was the time which made me more organized, more thoughtful and more sorted. I started valuing time more and started using my free time more judiciously. It gave me a chance to introspect and also gave me this glorious opportunity to reinvent myself. I reactivated my long lost hobby of writing which was hibernating under my busy work schedule all these days. I started penning down heartfelt stories which touched my soul and stirred my heart. I started observing the people around me more carefully, started talking to them more without being judgmental and started experiencing their lives from their point of view. The unique things I came across in my clinical practice, the smallest but sweet gesture of my little patients which made a huge impact on my mind inspired me to script these experiences as the eternal beautiful memories. Initially i started writing my experiences on my social media platform in my leisure time which was hugely appreciated and liked by many. Most of my family members and friends suggested that I should compile all these writings in a book so that it reaches to the larger massesand would benefit many.

So this marked the beginning of the making of Medical Miracles and after that I kept on writing continuously. The stories of kids with different aliments, their struggle to overcome the disease, the stories of courage and willpower to combat life's every odd and also the stories of Strong parents with their emotional journey… this book has it all. With lots of hard work and enormous efforts finally Medical Miracles is born. I have put my soul in these write-ups and have written each and every story with great love and affection. I hope many will get educated through my book and many parents will relate to the emotional turmoil radiating through these stories. I'm sure this book will take you on a roller coaster ride and you all will enjoy this journey filled with fun, laughter and tears as well.

So Dear Readers enjoy these write-ups, shower more love on me and do write to me how you felt reading my book. I will be more than happy to hear you out.

Lots of love and happiness always..........

Regards,

Dr. Pradnya. P. Wali.

DISCLAIMER

These stories are inspired by true events but are not the documentaries or biography of any characters depicted in this book. No scenes should be construed to represent a true or accurate recreation of the actual events that transpired. All the names, characters, places, location, events and incidents in this book are either the product of authors imagination or used in fictitious manner. Any resemblance of any character to actual persons, living or dead, or any resemblance of these stories to actual events is purely coincidental

CONTENTS

CHAPTER 1
AIRLIFT

"Baby is ready for being airlifted mam,we want you here urgent"message beeped on my cell.I urgently rushed to the ICU,did all the formalities and scrutinized stringently all the arrangements made for the baby with complicated liver disease to be shifted to Delhi for a rare and complex surgery. After an hour i got a call from our transport team that baby has been sucessfully airlifted and my mind and heart became suddenly light...as light as cottony sky. Atlast after 10 days of stormy course with that two months old baby with multiple problems of brain hemorrage; jaundice; blood infections,fits,a major brain surgery and ventilation we were finally able to pull out that baby to the stable state.Baby had complex liver problem requiring urgent surgery in the high end liver setup and so we have to take a call to transport this baby immediately.I relaxed in my chair sipping on the hot coffee and looking out from my favourite french window of my room.My heart and mind has already gone into the flashback by now as i recalled a similar incidence happened a few years back.

It's many years now but still each and every single moment

spent with that baby is fresh as dew. A two months old baby was admitted with recurrent lung infections from birth,was treated at multiple places,ventilated multiple times,has gulped doses and doses of antibiotics but still was not on the verge of recovery.Educated young smart couple walked in our counselling room with a web of worry on their forehead and lots of unasnwered questions in their eyes." We have come with lots of hope Doctor" mother said with the moist eyes.Yeah we will try our level best but we need to do some special test for your baby as we need to evaluate baby's problem completely i said assuringly.

Ok Doctor go ahead,do what so ever possible for my baby,father's husky baritone gave us the green signal.We did the detailed study of this baby's condition,took in depth history from the parents,did lots of discussions among our colleagues,browsed all the journals and research papers just to find out what more we can do for this baby as already this baby was investigated with multiple tests by many doctors of the various fields shopped by baby's parents and treated with almost all possible drugs.After lot of study we came to conclusion that work up for cystic fibrosis,Primary and Secondary immunodeficiency and IEM workup needs to be done. Parents were counselled in detail and the tests were sent.We all patiently waited for the results.

Everyday i used to look into the eyes of baby who was breathing on the ventilator trying to move all his limbs and waiting for the milk to be fed with his nasogastric tube.Those mysterious eyes used to give us the strength to work more for that young beating heart struggling to survive in this world.Cystic fibrosis and IEM workup is negative mam our resident doctor gave me the information.Ok so only one report awaited, trace immunodeficiency workup fast i reminded our doctors.Till then our laboratory incharge called up hurriedly telling that the reports have come and it was positive.I went into dizzy a bit as this was the last thing i wanted for my patient. I went through the report and it read as "Subacute Combined Immunodeficiency".My heart sank as i knew the only option for the treatment left was Bone marrow transplantation which was way too tedious requiring high end setup and more ever a matching donor.No doubt risk was high and chances were bleak but the parents were fighters as their baby was.Being a daughter of a Doctor herself,the mother and the father both were leaving no stone unturned to give the best possible treatment for their first born kid.We were explaining them the condition,treatment options,places where facilities were availble,risk; complications and prognosis involved.They too like a mature guardians were reading about the disease and were trying to understand the gravity of the situation. Meanwhile the baby's infection was controlled and he was extubated to the nasal prong oxygen.That alert look in his mysterious eyes always gave us hope to treat him.Baby was now on full feeds,his lungs showed signs of improvement and then parents came with the news that they have got the matching donor of one of the baby's sibling and they are ready for bone marrow transplant.

We appreciated their courage,their perseverance and dedication towards their child.We gave them the options where BMT could be done with the good results and they zeroed in on chennai as they had heard a lot about the institution there with high success rates for bone marrow transplantation.Parent flew to the chennai with all the reports and after going through the entire reports and current condition Doctors there gave us a green signal to shift the baby.Now the challenge was how to shift this baby to BMT centre.Road journey was quiet long requiring well equipped ambulance and Doctors to accompany them.After the in depth discussion with the family and friends they arranged for airlifting the baby.It was the shortest route by which baby would have landed in BMT centre quickly. Muliple trials were done successfully to test the lung compliance.Baby was breathing at ease even at room air but still i wasn't sure if this baby was fit to be airlifted with so much scarred lungs.Please arrange one doctor for us in the transport mam, will airlift the baby requested the parents.

After explaining the risk and complications which might occur mid air we arranged our doctor to accompany them and shifted the baby in the ambulance to the airport.Father bid farewell to the baby; mother and the baby's grandfather with heavy heart assuring them that he will reach chennai very soon.And here i was frequently reminding our Doctor to be alert.Flight took off going high and high up in the clouds.Father turned his car to go back and there was this sudden announcement of the emergency landing of the same flight on the Medical grounds.As the flight took off air pressure changes occured suddenly and baby lied pale and listless in the mother's lap.Our Doctor immediately rescucitated and intubated the baby in the air and was giving him breaths to count for his life.All the passengers were in total disbelief to what was happening.Unknowingly hundreds of them started praying in different languages,different manner together with only one good intention in their mind and heart requesting their respective Gods to shower the baby with new lease of life.

One could see a perfect example of unity in diversity in this critical situation.Father and emergency medical team at the airport rushed in to rescue the baby.Baby was breathing with a tube in his airways,heartbeat pounding.We are shifting the baby back to the hospital mam,baby collapsed midair crying father called at midnight.It was almost 2am past.We sent the hospital ambulance,retrieved the baby and put him back on the ventilator,his only life support helping him to breath to keep him alive. First time his mysterious alert eyes looked dim and dull to me.The chances are looking bleak i said softly to the parents.Next few days we did our level best on war foot to save the little life but sometimes your prayers go answered by Him.After days of struggling and fighting for the life the little warrior passed away.

The inconsolable cries of the parents kept resounding in my ears for long and this case got treasured deep in my heart.I saluted the little departed soul for his courage and fighting spirit.I saluted the strong and brave parents who did all their best possible efforts to save the young one.I could see the rainbow of emotions being a doctor.Every case can't be saved.No we are not Gods, we are the humans trained to save lives.We strive hard to make our patients relive the moments but cant give them additional brownie points of life more than designed by HIM,the Great Doctor and our Creator above.Days passed by and parents recuperated but they always kept the gratitude towards us for all the support we extended and all the trials we gave. They could sense the deep efforts we made for their baby. Most of the times moral and emotional support is needed along with the medical support.Parents went along with the flow of time,got busy in their daily lives posting their family pictures and sending their notes of well being intermittently to us.Really your patients sometime becomes your extended families.These bonds are more emotional and trustful.We are planning for our next baby mam and we are getting all our antenatal genetic tests done read my FB message one fine day.A smile flashed on my face and my morning felt to be much brighter than the bright sun outside."All the best guys..i wish you all the life's very best and i'm sure you will enjoy parenthood healthier this time", i replied.The tears rolled down my cheeks all mixed with joy,happiness,curiosity and prayers for them.

As someone knocked on my room door i came out of my flashback.Mam baby has safely reached the capital and they are planning for the surgery tomorrow my junior told me with a smile. I heaved a sigh of relief atlast a succesful airlifting finally this time.Good job done guys,keep it up !! I appreciated my team effort and moved to my next patient positively.Really this Medical life makes you to live hundred of lives in one.And we relive a new life with every life we save!!

* * *

CHAPTER 2

BILLA NO: 420

After a refreshing and rejuvenating Dubai trip i checked into the Dubai airport. Done with my immigration and Airport formalities I relaxed down in the Magestic Rocking Sofa just like His Highness of Dubai Emperor waiting for my flight boarding announcement to be done.Yet my mind was still whirling around in the miraculous Miracle Garden of Dubai, Glittering Global Village and my heart dancing on the tunes of Bollywood music at the Bollywood park of Dubai which I had recently visited.Ohhh you cannot have enough of Dubai in one go..! I was just sitting and recalling the thrilling moments of the New year celebrated at Burj Khalifa when i got a soft voice disturbing my thoughts "Hello mam; how are you.?" I was amazed to see someone recognising me at the distant land.I gave a fresh smile and reverted back I'm all good, how are you? I'm fine mam but did you recognise me? She asked with the same silent smile on her face.Her popped up cheek bones, upfronted teeth, broad nose looked familiar but my brain was too lazy to come out of the rosy thoughts of my recent trip to remind me who this young lady in her early 20 was! I nodded in a big No and she said with a soft smile"I'm Billa no 420"GMC Miraj".

I was suddenly shocked and surprised.My eyes were button big and my brows went a few inches high.Suddenly it took me 10 years back when i have just finished my Pediatric post graduation and was working in the Government Medical college.We used to have these myriad of patients here of different varieties and treating them used to be a new challenge everyday.Sitting in the OPD on a busy Wednesday afternoon i called out next patient.Someone walked slowly and got sitted onto the chair. Yes plz tell me i said without lifting my head to see who was next on the patient's chair. Hb is 5 gm blood transfusion day today,need your signature on this a soft,tender voice banged on my ear. I saw it curiously only to find a very small girl who may be 10 years old with a slip in her hand sitting on the front chair in a calm and composed way.Who are you? i asked her with a smile.I'm Billa no 420 Thalassemia unit she said.I was so amused to hear that. Who has accompanied you? my next question.No i have come alone.Every month i come here by myself.Parents work as coolie in other's farm.They can't afford to accompany me everytime wasting their money and morever i know the procedure here she said firmly.I was in awe of her bravery.

True...many old and young chronic patients in government hospitals cannot afford to get accompanying persons as they work on daily wages.We have this big Thalassemia ward in the government hospital which caters to these Thalassemia patients and take care of their monthly blood transfusions.Thalassemia is a genetic disorder of blood formation which needs blood transfusion every 20-30 days and it runs in the families.I signed her paper and she went to the ward,got her blood transfusion done and waved me bye bye while going back to her home.

Next week i saw her again in my OPD.I asked her confusingly your transfusion is over last week only why have you come back again today.Cold? Cough? Fever?? She said smilingly no mam nothing for me this time, it's my brother's blood transfusion today,his Hb is 6 gms.And behind her came her 6 yrs old fragile,weak brother trailing her frock.I was shocked as it was B Thalassemia Major where in she and her brother both had got this disease.I felt soo sad.So you get him every month here? i asked her.Yes mam i get him on Saturdays usually so both of us won't miss our schools she updated me.She took my sign on the blood requisition form and took him to Thalassemia ward for his transfusion.I felt soo sorry for both of them.What a life i whispered to myself.They are Avani and Aakash who come here ever month madam for blood transfusion.Our Thalassemia patients on record, both are very obedient and co operative.Entire department and Thalassemia unit people knows them here our OPD incharge Asha sister told me while keeping hot tea cup in front of me.

I finished my busy OPD and started for my home.Walking in the corridor my heart was so heavy and unknowingly my feet turned towards Thalassemia ward.Let me have a look at them before i go; I thought to myself as i reached the ward. The younger boy was getting transfused and only little blood was left.No pain,no agonies,no suffering on their face.Elder girl,his Tai was talking to him and feeding him parle G biscuits.Both were laughing and were busy in their own small world. I was amazed to see their courage to fight life's every odd with such a great brave face. So...what you two are doing? i interrupted them.Nothing mam i'm diverting him so that he will forget his i.v line pain she said smilingly.You guys aren't afraid of this iv cannula, blood transfusion every month? I asked them painfully. Mam,we are born with this so whether to sit and crib or embrace and learn to live with this is our choice.We take transfusion and go back and do our normal routine work as if nothing has happened.We don't even feel we have got any kind of disease she said affirmatively.I was shocked with their so much positivity about the life.There are many great things we learn from these small innocent faces.Their little words of wisdom have power to change one's World.

From then every month i started meeting them.I used to buy them biscuits and fruits every time I met them and talked about every aspect of life.Our conversations used to be very intresting including stories of great people and how they conquered their illness to small daily routines from their school.I was trying to motivate them and make them more strong to face their illness but some where deep i knew they were radiating their positivity on me.Days passed i left GMC for my Superspeciality fellowship and life went on. These small brother and sister were left behind in my thoughts.And suddenly today on the Dubai airport I met this young girl calling herself Billa no 420!

I enquired about her well being. Mam I fared well in my 10 th and 12 th board exams and now working in MNC she told. Along with my job I'm working as educator for Thalassemic patients.I'm creating awareness among the public about this disease, motivating them for screening and supporting families with this disease and helping them to get monthly transfusions.I'm working at Mumbai and have come here for Thalassemia Awareness talk.I felt soo happy seeing my young patients turning out to be so dynamic and doing so good! We only treat these small children but they were healing this World in the true sense.

I said well done my Bravo! I'm proud of you.Keep up the good work going. She bought me a hot cup of coffee,opened her purse and took out the same Parle G biscuits i used to offer her everytime.I took 1-2 biscuits with a hearty laugh."Taste bhi - Health bhi : Parle G....tin tin tidin..." We chanted in chorus. It was our mantra back in GMC days in Thalessemia ward. These brave kids are more miraculous than Miracle garden i thought.I felt like I got my return gift today!

* * *

CHAPTER 3

THE INTOUCHABLES

Three of us boarded the cab early in the morning.It was still quite dark and silent outside.This was an important day of the year for me as every year on this day i go to remote areas where poor and needy people belong to and serve them.It's my granny's death anniversary and I'm doing it without fail in her loving memory for years now.So this year we had planned a visit to an Orphanage but not only to feed and donate them some essential things but morsoever to educate them.

When i was thinking where should I heed this year my staff nurse gave me a clue about this orphanage. It was an all girls orphanage with around 60 of them between 10-16 years and this very thought struck me why not educate them on the most under rated and less talked topic of Menstrual Hygiene.I did my homework, made a small Audio-visual PowerPoint presentation, took the school stationary, books and sweets to distribute and left my house in the early wee hour to reach this place.We had called the orphanage rector who was all set to prepare a hearty meal for all the children on behalf of us.

Our cab started making its way from the rough roads and

narrow paths full of pebbles and ditches.Both sides were green farmlands and small huts standing and bending on each other. Looks like a small habitat i thought to myself.Women were draped in the clothes covering them from head to toe and there was this small window like opening on their face covering pardah near to their eyes just to see the outer world.No doubt it was the most underdeveloped areas with no contact with today's modern World.Our cab stood still near the old shattered gate. I along with two of my senior nurses got down with our boxes of eatables,stationary and then pushed the broken gate.It went on making sound as if it was waiting for its oiling for ages now. May be it was their door bell because instantly two middle-aged women came forward and took the boxes from our hands. One was the rector and the incharge of this orphanage and other one was their Cook. We started walking behind them.It was a very old dilapidated building with washed off colour, broken stairs and wretched walls.Crossing over the small-small rooms by side of passage(may be this was where those girls stayed) we entered a big hall.They have tried to make it look neat with a big cloth spread on the ground.One old table with clean white table cloth was kept in middle of the room with a glass flowerpot standing tall.Colourful flowers were the only colourful thing in that room.Girls in their early teens from 10-14 years were sitting close to each other with the fear, anxiety and curiosity flowing on their faces.

We took out our projector and board and our nurses started fixing it. I started my laptop and opened my presentation.So girls...shall we start ?I asked them enthusiastically. But the scared girls didn't reply.They were seeing stealthily from the angle of their eyes to my Lucknowi dress with thread work embedded with glass, long oxidised zhumkas in my ear and my inherant confidence.Then they stared at our two nurses dressed in their uniforms with neatly bunned hair and their white rectangular cap pinned up in their hair which was something very new and strange to them. They haven't seen women so secure yet independent like this. I knew it was the time to relax them.I went and sat between them and told i was here to show them a movie.A movie to which they all will relate and as i started the documentary on menstrual hygiene there was this loud scary scream among them.....shiiiiii.....what is this.....ammo...they put their hands on their mouth in shock and closed their eyes. Older girls started giggling about what these people were showing us and they started shoving off the young girls out of the room saying you go off from here it's not for you.

I was shocked and stunned. Still so much stigma and taboo around this topic? Are we really in the 21st century I wondered. I calmed the girls and told them there was nothing to havoc. It's natural to have periods and the menstrual cycle is a part of our reproductive system.We being women should be proud that we are blessed by Mother Nature with the ability of giving birth to someone like us creating our own mirror image.And again which is the boon only we women have got. We are the creators,we are the nurturors and this superpower only and only we women have got! So we all are superwomen!! Now listening to this they got bit attentive, their weirdness and anxiety reduced and they were now mentally prepared to watch the documentary.I educated them about the importance of menstrual cycle,the changes which girls go through from their childhood to adolescence, the role of hormones in our body and how to accept this gracefully.And then we spoke and spoke about mood changes, behavioural changes, pain and aches, slow flow and heavy flow and measures to tackle this pains and mood swings.By the end of talk every girl looked motivated and was actively participating in the topic discussion.They were no more shy and timid girls which i saw an hour back but they all looked so enlightened! After my talk many came forward and were discussing their period aliments.All were common issues and needed only reassurance. I prescribed a few medicines for their PMS and cramps.I told them the importance of hygiene during these days,the role of a good diet and moderate exercise.Girls were now looking more confident after gaining knowledge about their monthly issues.Now they knew nothing was bad blood, no need to sit separately in a corner during those days, no need to eat alone, no need to sleep in the dark and on damp floors like intouchables and morsoever no need to behave different.My talk made them to believe themselves as Normal and realised that they carry a boon of motherhood in their womb contrary to what they were told that they bleed because they are evil spirits and are cursed.It was much important to get them out of this illogical and senseless thoughts which were imbibed in them from their births.It was not so easy for them to come out of their cocoon and spread their wings but these girls atleast tried to dare that. I was glad that i could spread some light on this much tabood topic and could break the glass ceiling and make them believe that they are actually not the intouchables!!!

Hot hot meal was ready by now.We all sat together on the warm blankets spread on the ground.There were no issues about impure blood and evil spirits,there were no issues about red dot and red panda now.Having a hearty meal together made us all human but more so over the wonderful women that we were!!

* * *

CHAPTER 4

TRAIN TO RAJASTHAN

Numaish...the word only brings so much joy on our faces.This word is emotion to every Hyderabadi! Yes we all Hyderabadis will be waiting year long to roam, eat and shop in this exhibition stalls.Numaish in Urdu is exhibition and this Grand Annual Exhibition is a treat for every shopping lover to get the exclusive things across the country.There are Kashmiri stalls with their hallmark pashmina shawls and stoles, Lucknowi Kurtis with thread and glass work,fine cutlery and crockery, Rajasthani jewellery with big round kada kangan, long ear pieces, oxidised zhumkas, mirror work lehenga choli and not to miss the tasty vegetarian and non-vegetarian big eateries to savouir your hungry tounge.Being an art and fashion lover I will be vrroming in this Numaish every year on full shopping spree..!

Numaish...it's like a sea of people.. lakhs in number roaming and enjoying the festive vibes here. I remember the Jatra of my home town where we all the kids,elders and teenagers used to go and enjoy the giant wheel rounds and panipuri,chats and bhel on the roadside stalls.Likewise this year i was enjoying the joy ride in this exclusive flea market of Numaish purchasing things of my choice when i could feel someone pulling my dress from behind. I turned in astonishment only to find a small 4 year old boy wearing jeans and red t-shirt and big matching red hat paired with Goggles trying to seek my attention.The moment I turned around he started shouting " yeh meri doctor hai, yeh meri doctor hai",hearing his loud tone his mother came out rushing from the shopping crowd and looking at each other we started smiling. Yes he was right i was his doctor and he was my chotu patient Vansh whom I was seeing from day 1 of his life.

His mother Richa had high risk pregnancy and hence this baby was delivered and got shifted to my special care unit.The joy of holding him in her hands after losing her 3 babies was immeasurable..!! He was 3.3 kgs healthy baby and was kept in the ICU for minor breathing issue and for the monitoring of blood sugars as the mother had high level of sugars during her pregnancy.After initial see-saw phase in Nicu we handed him to his mother on the 4th day.She took some time to learn handling him and feeding.Our Lactation counsellor helped her to reduce her anxiety and taught her various positions of breastfeeding so that the mother can be at ease.Richa's mother helped her to take care of him.On the day of discharge they got big packets of Namkeen, Bhujiya Sev and tins of Rasgulla for me as a token of appreciation.Wow So many Delicacies i exclaimed.We produce our own items Mam we have factory of these items at the outskirts of the city.We do manufacture,packaging and sell as well they updated me.Now eating all these sweet savouirs daily Vansh will be more healthier i said to them and then mother-daughter duo bursted out laughing.

She came regularly for the follow - up visits to me and for monthly Vaccinations.She always appreciated that my technique of vaccination is awesome and vansh never gets any pain or fever after the injections.He is all normal, eating and playing after all the jabs.What more a mother needs than her child playing and happy all the times after getting injections she used to say. Time flew and he was 5 months old.Mam can I take him and travel now? she asked me at one of his regular visit.where are you going? I enquired. Rajasthan mam, my in-laws place she updated me.Ohhh where in Rajasthan?? Jalore district she added.Yeah you can but be careful in travelling. I gave her tips as how to travel with the baby and then they went to Rajasthan but kept coming every month or two for the baby's check ups with me. Their train to and fro from Rajasthan was always booked.Why you travelling from so far? You can consult a pediatrician there itself I said her.No mam, you have magic in your hands.The day since he is born you are seeing him.You know what suits him better, he never cries out of pain after your injections.I have this positive feeling with you.I will keep coming to you only mam.That way I can meet my mother as well she smiled.Ohh two birds in one shot i trolled her and we both smiled.

In his every visit to Hyderabad Vansh kept visiting me atleast once or twice.when he was a year old his mother brought him with wheezing complaint.They have roamed all over their city in Rajasthan meeting many doctors but couldn't get relief. So as soon as she landed in Hyderabad they came to me the very next day. I could even feel his wheeze while holding him and walking upstairs and downstairs she said.He was otherwise well but had wheeze associated respiratory infection.Do anyone at home has allergy or asthma? i enquired. Yes his paternal grandfather has asthma, uses nebulizer intermittently she informed. I wrote medicines and nebulizations and told her if frequent episodes occur he may require Huff Puff kit as it can lead to childhood Asthma.But even to my surprise he was completely alright after 3 days of medicines and those symptoms never recurred in him again till date and their faith in me increased leaps and bounds.I have seen him from sparse hair to pony tail of his hair to hairstyle of dashing Rock star. Really you can witness few kids literally growing in front of you.And today he was here in the Numaish with hunky funky dress and Goggles calling me his Doctor. The surrounding was lit with grand lightings and flock of men and women were chirping around in their colourful clothes making exhibition more vibrant.I bought him big blue balloon with red lights inside which were glittering high. Little Vansh was overjoyed to see it and started dancing on the tunes of Bollywood music playing on the loudspeaker nearby. The happiness of the kids is so inexpensive in all the ways i thought. They find happiness in every small things.We need to learn this art of finding happiness in small things from them.We will come to meet you in two days mam, his mother told me.Ohh anytime..i smiled. So their train to Rajasthan had some time still i smiled to myself and started walking.There was now more life to this unknown crowd around me!

* * *

CHAPTER 5
BUBBLE MUM

"I want to see the doctor urgently"...a well groomed, well dressed woman in her early 30's came to the reception hurriedly breaking the patient line and started yelling in loud voice.Who is the patient mam? What has happened? My soft spoken receptionist Mrudula asked her in a gentle tone. She was indeed like her name Mrudula...gentle,sweet,soft spoken lady with a charming face and warm smile. You aren't Doctor so why I should tell you? just send me inside, its urgent.She pushed the man in front of her and made herself way to the reception counter. Where is your child mam ? Tell me baby's name my receptionist asked her to register the patient.There he is, she pointed to the sitting arena. A chubby child of about two and a half year was sitting on the bench eating ice candy and looking happy. So is he the patient? my receptionist asked in a subtle way.Yes can't you see he is so sick and unwell? send me inside right now she spoke angrily. Mam other patients are waiting from long, can you wait for a while till then I'll make his card? Mrudula told her.Cant you hear? my child is so sick, he has high fever that's why i have given him ice candy to cool him down. It's dire emergency she banged her Gucci bag on the counter,her lipstick got bit spread as she screamed. I was seeing this altercation on the CCTV screen in my cabin. I called on the reception and told to send her inside.

She came hurriedly inside banging the door pulling her child.His one shoe flung into the air as she dragged him inside the door. Your Reception people are the worst madam, they can't understand the importance of emergency. I was trying to make them understand that my baby is so sick but they weren't letting me in.They wasted my precious 10 minutes she said furiously looking at her costly stone studded watch.She was chubby, fair, tall lady in pricey salwar suit with properly manicured hands,long red painted nails,

iPhone in one hand, a Gucci bag on the other hand and a branded watch on the wrist.She looked affluent and arrogant. I didn't wanted to drag this conversation so i came straight to the point.Please have a sit, would you like to have some water? I tried to cool her down. She drank water hastily from the glass kept on my table. Thanks doctor, I drink only black mineral water at home but as you offered i drank it now.See my child he is having high grade fever since yesterday she continued. I examined the child and everything seemed to be okay. His temperature was normal and vitals stable. May be its just environmental fever,nothing much serious i told her.No doctor we stay indoors always in full AC, hardly go out in the sun, if we want to step out we go in fully AC car so how can he get environmental fever? she was in the denial mode.Okay I see may be some viral fever but other signs aren't there of viral etiology. Anyways I'm writing paracetamol so when he gets fever just give him the dose I tried explaining her. What paracetamol?? Doctor I can buy it from pharmacist as well.For that i need not waste my time here.My child is so sick you write him some good antibiotics she insisted. I don't advise antibiotics for simple fever. He is stable and not even having fever now so you can give him this syrup only when he gets fever i handed her my prescription.That next lane Doctor always write good antibiotics so fever subsidies early. Why can't you write too? You Doctors want us to visit you again and again so you don't write everything at one go she started again. I said look Madam, antibiotics has to be used judiciously and have certain indications to prescribe. Antibiotics wont work for viral fever. Unnecessary usage of antibiotics causes more harm than good to the child.Once he develops resistance to the antibiotics it will be difficult to treat further infections then.Give this paracetamol syrup for 2-3 days even then if fever remains high grade or child develops cold,cough or other symptoms get him back. I tried explaining her rationality of the antibiotic usage. But all in vain she left annoyed and did not turn back for almost a week.

Again a week later I could hear the same noise at the reception counter. The same lady has come with her child with a small juice can holding in his hand. She argued and argued but my receptionist patiently handled her this time and sent her inside only on her turn. How is your child now? i asked her.You didn't write any antibiotics doctor, his fever won't subside without antibiotics. So i went to next lane doctor the same day and got some antibiotics. But he developed loose motions.So i went to him again and he wrote different antibiotic. Now his loose motions have stopped but he is vomiting continuously she dumped prescription of the other doctor in front of me. Prescription of oral Amoxicillin has led to loose motions, to control that another antibiotic was given which has put child into gastritis leading to vomitings. I examined him thoroughly. He was absolutely stable and well hydrated. There wasn't any signs of dehydration. But had some uneasy feeling in epigastric region and nausea. I told her to stop all the antibiotics and prescribed some simple antiemetic,antacid and symptomatic treatment. What stop antibiotics? Then how his infection will be cured doctor? She asked disappointedly. Unnecessary antibiotics is causing him this all problems I tried explaining but this time i cut it short. By now i knew she will go on doctor shopping and enter another clinic to force write some antibiotic for her satisfaction.

Next week again she was here in my cabin with urine container holding in her hand. Madam my child is very sick.I think he has got jaundice. He is passing yellow coloured urine since two days and she showed me the urine what she has collected. Yes it was indeed high coloured. I sent it for urine analysis which was normal. No bile salts or bile pigments noted in the urine. Child didn't had jaundice clinically also.Liver function tests were normal as well. I told them it might be due to dehydration and told her to give plenty of water and free fluids.Why won't you admit and treat him? Give him some iv fluids and iv injections, don't worry about money.My child's health is most important she kept on stressing. I know you are the mother and naturally worried about your child. But as of now he looks okay to me.If needed i will surely admit and treat I assured her. She left reluctantly disappointed.

After 15-20 days again she entered my opd this time looking rather anxious. What happened now? I asked her. He is passing blood in his motions she told as she put his diaper in front of me. There was this some blood stain on the diaper.I examined the child and local area very carefully but everything looked normal again.No history of constipation. I advised to keep him in the hospital this time for observation and sent his stool for laboratory check.Yes there was blood in the stool in report as well. I started thinking child looks normal, stool consistency normal, local examination normal then from where the blood is coming. I kept him in the ward under strict nursing monitoring and blood never appeared in the stools for next 2 days. Ultrasound abdomen also didn't reveal anything significant either. Child was eating well and hence we shifted him to the room with his mother. And again to our dismay in the afternoon the child had blood in the stool.Mother came running to my opd showing his diaper having few stains of fresh blood. I went to his room and found the child sitting peacefully on the bed and playing with his soft toy.Now my brain started working in the other way. My neuronal anttenas stood straight as I thought of something else and shifted the child to the special room.We counselled her as this room was near to the nursing station she could get their help immediately if she needed so she

I was sure will crack this diagnosis shortly. I kept a watch on her and the child through the CCTV. I told my nurse in charge and IT department people to closely monitor them.This room had cctv surveillance and in no time our sister came running and said "yes madam you were right when the child passes motion she is pricking her finger with pin and adding few blood drops on to the diaper.I have told IT department person to get that clip here." But how did you get on to this diagnosis?she asked me curiously. I smiled and said sixth sense. Initially when she came I thought she is arrogant and over protective mother who is hyper anxious about her child.Many parents do insist for the antibiotics and even purchase it over the counter and treat their child.They think each and every sickness is cured only by the antibiotics. But this lady kept coming repeatedly with different complaints and everytime child looked normal without any medical issue.Her behaviour showed she was anxious and psychologically disturbed. She always spoke high about herself and how she and her husband splurged on exotic things but deep inside she was sad and unhappy.

Last time when she was showing me the diaper I could see few prick marks on her fingers and that time only i clicked this case. When i asked her about those prick marks she told she has high sugar so she keeps checking her sugar levels regularly. But i was pretty sure that it's a case of Manchausen by proxy means here child doesn't have any physical illness but parent or child keep exaggerating it due to mental stress,strain and other psychological issues.Last time also when she came with the complaint of high coloured urine, urine was very yellow to view but urine analysis was normal, liver functions were normal and child didn't had any visible jaundice. In my opd when I was examining the baby,he peed and it was normal urine but when she brought the urine in the urine container it was deep yellow and i could smell strong pungent multivitamin odour to it and I was pretty sure that she has added few drops of multivitamin drops to it. But as we didn't had any evidence i just let her go. So this time i insisted them to stay in the special room with CCTV coverage so that we can crack this case and come to the diagnosis which we did effectively. All our staff were numb to hear this story. Psychological issues are on rise than physical illness in this era.

Here mother requires treatment and not the child I told our staff. We called our phyciatrist and counselled her. She accepted the fact that she did it to come out of her house. Her husband was a big businessman and extremely busy. He travelled a lot and wasn't able to give her any time. They belonged to highly conservative family and she wasn't allowed to step out of her home for anything.There was no one to talk or share. Old in-laws needed care and her entire time was going into monitoring the kitchen and routine chores and taking care of her in-laws. In the earlier days she spent like crazy on shopping branded dresses, watches, bags and parlour. Monthly kitties were arranged at her home with lavish meals and drinks. But soon she started getting bored of living this artificial life.People used to come, enjoy the expensive spread of variety of dishes and leave but she couldn't find any real person to share and care. She started feeling extremely lonely and then she built a virtual world around her and started staying in her own bubble. She used to talk to herself and was acting as if she is going for outings,movies,hotels with her husband and kept boasting about those virtual things to the people around her. She bought few expensive things for self satisfaction. And when she didn't find any reason to step out of her house she started making excuses of the child's health and started visiting hospitals again and again. She started asking for antibiotics to stress the seriousness of illness so that she can be with her child and escape from the house chores. She wanted to be in the hospital so that she can be away from her daily routine for 2- 3 days and her husband could spare some time for them.

In short she was very much stressed out emotionally and mentally exhausted. We called her husband and counselled him. He was surprised to know her condition and assured us he will spare time for her and his son. Living under the same roof he wasn't aware what his wife was going through.He always thought he is providing her every luxurious thing so she may be happy but here he forgot that the most precious thing what one need is love ,care,affection and most importantly the time of their loved ones.They deployed extra care takers for their old in laws.She underwent therapy and was started on the medications.

Her husband started spending time with her and his son.They started having family lunch together. Eventually her in laws health also started getting better and they looked more healthy. Slowly she improved and looked more happy and cheerful now.Her visit to my hospital became almost nil. Although i was short by one patient now i was happy that she could improve and bounce back to normalcy. All the illness do not require medicines always. Most of the time and almost everytime they require TLC....i.e. Tender, Love, care. In this busy hustly bustly life we are forgetting the basic things needed for our mental well being. It's very important to spend time with the family and friends to keep our mind and heart happy.Loving unconditionally and Hearty laugh are the two powerful medicines which keeps most of the aliments at bay. So be happy and keep smiling always. Simple joys in our lives makes it more beautiful and worth living.Simple vitamin of Vitamin H i.e vitamin Happiness is the cure for most of our things.Everything cannot be bought or counted in money at last.Finally i was glad that I could break this virtual bubble of this mother staying in the bubble world and bring her back to the reality.

* * *

CHAPTER 6

A GIRL IN THE YELLOW BOOTS

Tuk tuk tuk gentle knock and my consultation room door opened slowly and some soft sound of walking in those Hallmark yellow cute little boots sensed me that SHE is coming !! This is for you….a fresh bright yellow rose she kept on my table trying to pull herself climb on the front chair and sit.Mam these sweets are for you, her mother Radha opened the peda box in front of me and smiled.Ohh what's special? sweets and all today I asked. She got First rank in the District level drawing competition her mother told proudly with a twinkle in her eyes.This girl in the yellow boots took out a nice drawing of a lady sitting on the table and chair with her proud possession of stethescope around her neck. That's for you…..it's you she said with a broad smile.I was amused to see my caricature drawn in a very finer way.Ohhh so this is me right? I asked laughing out loud.It's very pretty, absolutely amazing I admired her drawing skills.Yes..just like you!she told me looking farther out from my room's window. She drew it last night mam, her mother added with the same twinkle in her eyes.Those twinkle in her eyes said it all!

Prerna was her name but her fondness for the yellow and her

all time favourite yellow boots which drew my attention instantly with lights shimmering from the sides of those boots tempted me to name her as "the girl in the yellow boots!".She was a special child around 5 years old now. Survival of the fittest was the term applied to her in every sense.Born with a severe tracheal stenosis (severe narrowing of the wind pipe by birth) she was brought with severe breathing difficulty to our Nicu at the midnight past. I still remember that thrilling night when I got a call from our Nicu resident about her case and I rushed out immediately to attend her.In emergency every second counts.She was lying pale in the warmer with severe distress fighting for the life.Every breath pumped through the artificial support system via bag and mask helped her to hold on.

Intubation failed mam, my resident told in a panicky mode.I inserted the larnyngoscope only to find a very small,almost pea sized tracheal opening.She has got a very severe tracheal stenosis we wont be able to intubate her I said grimly.What's next now? my resident asked sweating profusely baging the baby beneath the warmer.Only option is Emergency Tracheostomy i said.But who will come this late at night and that to for bedside Tracheostomy in such a small baby? he asked me worriedly. Let me try I said thoughtfully.It was almost 2am in the night when we ringed our Ent surgeon.Deep in his sleep he heard about the case,got up shockingly and rushed immediately knowing the seriousness of the baby's condition.Here the doctors were doing everything on the war foot to save the child but sometimes attenders/ relatives are so cold to understand the importance of any emergency.

We counselled the attenders regarding the airway problem and briefed them about the need of emergency Tracheostomy (making a hole in the windpipe) to help her breath.Attenders were confused and equally anxious.Their minds went blank and they weren't in the position to decide.Father started arguing with maternal relatives that he had no money to spend on such a defective child and fleeted from the scene saying he doesn't want that baby.Attenders were in two thoughts whether to treat or not.Female baby,in future if she will have problems then it would be difficult.Leave it madam will take her to government hospital maternal uncle's were saying annoyingly. Maternal grandmother was crying aloud as to why the very first child of her daughter was born like this questioning the very own existence of the God.But only mother was firm and unshaken.I want my child at any cost.Do whatever possible madam but save her she was repeatedly telling on phone. I told the attenders it's a dire emergency and we cannot waste time like this and they have to take some decision instantly. Finally on the mother's insistence, uncle's gave in on their reluctance and gave their consent for this procedure.

Our Ent surgeon, a old Punjabi doctor, tall, sturdy with long white beard and his turban reached our Nicu on his Bajaj scooter.This was his pride possession which he didn't wanted to give off. He always felt in the emergency his scooter will take him faster on those busy roads making way through the crowd rather than any A.C four wheeler. He was ready with his scrubs on and six steps of hand washing. I looked at these two heros of that night, one our Nicu resident who was literally drenching in the sweat standing below the radiant warmer but didn't give up pumping the oxygen to the baby and then was this old Punjabi man who came in no time at this odd hours to save this unknown life. Both looked like a knighthood in their shining armour to me.Emergency Tracheostomy was done bedside and baby was connected to the ventilator. Finally all the thrill and anxiety decreased when we could see the child breathing smoothly on the ventilator and her vitals getting stabilised. When the whole world was busy asleep tight in the dark night we few people were struggling hard applying all our skill and knowledge to save some life! We waited for an hour for the things to get settled. Repeat ABG was far better.We counselled the attenders post procedure, showed them their baby and settled in our chairs when the clock strucked four am. Hot steamy tea relaxed the tension which our brains carried so long. We spoke about these various emergency scenarios which we have come across in our practice. Our Punjabi surgeon told how he did tracheostomy on 130 kgs hefty man with a very short neck and then on this small baby hardly weighing 2.5 kgs on the same day!For the Doctors like us busy Saving lives we have always many stories to tell.I thanked our Ent surgeon for his timely intervention as he left.I could see the sky turning crimson from mauve and the rays of rising sun made the atmosphere more warm and optimistic.Many a times our hospital and Nicu are our homes. We eat,we work and spend most of our times here. The satisfaction on our faces of the job done well was just so perfect…just like a picture to frame!

Days went on…The baby improved and was weaned off from ventilator. Mother was trained in the Tracheostomy tube care and then discharged. She kept on coming for follow ups,vaccinations and never missed a single checkup.All on her own.Her husband abandoned her, her own family members denied any more financial help stating their own personal reasons. Finally everyone will have their life and problems to deal and family to feed. But nothing can ever deter mother's courage and determination.Every mother's sacrifice and strong will power will always find a way out for her child.Especially the mother of this child was really brave to take this decision and raise her child single-handedly.Looking at ladies like her I realised why our women are called as Maa Durga, Chandi, Kali, Mahalakshmi and so on.Really the courage, the power, the efforts a mother puts for her child determinantly no one ever on this earth can do! The baby had stiffness of the muscles making her development bit slow.It was the result of decreased oxygen supply to brain due to her stormy neonatal course. I referred her to a good physiotherapist for early stimulation and intervention.

She kept on coming to me every now and then following every instructions of mine very religiously.Slowly the baby improved albiet with some developmental delay.But she was now able to walk and talk in her baritone voice because of tracheostomy closure. She was bit slow in learning as compared to her peers but she was born with that "Never give up Attitude" like her mother.She enjoyed going to her special school and learning new skills daily.Whenever she visited me she made me laugh heartily with her school stories and jokes.Her puffed up face,big eyes,out turned lips were left far behind and her happy glowing face made her look more beautiful to me.Yeah she was slow but yet so special.And that specialness overflowed through the eyes of her proud mother.

What should I name her mam? Prerna?? Is that name ok? She asked me one day.Yeah very relevant name go ahead I said happily. Prerna means positive energy, Prerna means inspiration and this girl and her mother were indeed the true inspiration for this whole materialistic world which works only on give and take buisness.The love between this mother and child was so pure and powerful beyond any gains, profits or any returns. It was selfless and so it was divine. Today's this prize of this special girl for her drawing skill was a slap for the entire male dominated earth who always understated girls and their calibre to excel. Soo that's the story of this girl in yellow boots.Her consultation was over and she walked out with her mother holding her finger tight.Lights emitting out of her magical shoes were making my room more radiant,vibrant and bright!!!!!

* * *

CHAPTER 7

FINDING NEVERLAND

Can you please come home and talk to Rishab once? Nisha my childhood friend on the other side of the call was requesting me in a very sobby tone.Something wrong again my internal voice told me.It wasn't very convenient to ask her details on the phone in a busy OPD of mine.Yeah I'll come in the evening i assured her.I wrapped up my OPD early and reached Nisha's home by 6 pm.She was sitting on the chair in hall all worried, her face was grumpy telling that she was crying since morning,her hair were unkempt indicating something major has happened.I patted her back, went into the kitchen, made some coffee and brought two mugs outside, " have it and you will feel better" i said as i offered her coffee.She fell on my shoulders and started crying.He is getting out of control, getting violent for small things,go look at his room everything precious in the room he has broken today i don't know what should I do and she broke down!! I consoled her, made her to have some coffee and assured her i'll talk to him. I can only console, her pain only she can feel...after all she was a mother.

. . .

I walked to his room and pushed his half opened door he was sitting on his rolling chair with his mobile playing some game. His face was red and he looked angry.Rishab was teenage boy of my childhood friend,her parents and mine were neighbours for more than 6 decades. Rishabh was a smart and intelligent guy of generation Z,Net savy and tech savvy with great minds in the computers.He was well read and had good knowledge about the current affairs and international politics but he was very reserved, person of few words and few friends.He never mingled with his peers and never had a hearty laugh.Either he was busy with studies orelse surfing on the net,Netflix series and seasons were his only world.I have seen him growing in front of me.

Nisha and Amit both were too intelligent and were on the higher posts in MNC's. Both drew handsome salary and they all led hifi life with no dearth of anything.They loved their son to core but expected him to fare very well and succeed in his life as they did and were providing him with every comfort which they couldn't afford. I went to him and said a soft hi...! He looked at me,didn't react and again put his neck into his mobile.So you don't want to talk to your friend today i poked him.I don't want to speak to anyone what's there to speak he said arrogantly.Accha so if you don't want to speak to me let's speak to our phone only then i too will play pub G.After all i drove 12 kms in heavy traffic to play pub G only na here i said.. he mellowed down a bit.Why are you so rude to your mother? I asked.And why they both are rude to me?? he questioned me back.They are your parents Rishab, she is your mother! I tried explaining.Yeah yeah I know Remote mummy, scolding Daddy and Robot son...he whimed.What?i asked shockingly.

Yes I'm their robot son.My mother has my remote, she presses button and i have to get up, rishab it's 6 am get up, 6.15 brush your teeth, 6.30- start studying....rishab eat this,this is healthy, rishab wear this it looks good on you, rishab do that, rishab don't do that, rishab dont go there, why you want to go to a movie? You will be wasting so much time...in that span you will cover your algebra lesson and then there's my scolding dad,Rishabh don't roam with your useless friends after classes...you have to prepare for IAS, I'm spending so much on your tutions, books, don't let me down. Always they dictate and i follow like a robot.Don't i have any feelings and decisions of mine?I'm feeling choked. Granny understands everything but whenever she tries to speak they both warn her not to interfere as it's my future ka sawal and then she is like a mute spectator. Arre but why they don't understand...for my future i should live my present first he was furious and ranting continuously. I have no liberty,no choices and no decision making here.Is it my home or jail ??? And he started crying.For the very first time i was seeing him speaking so much, the very reserved kid of all times was trying to vent out his frustration and anger.I tried him to calm down. The neck throttling competition of today's world and parental pressure to achieve everything in one shot was taking a toll on his body and mind. In such situations many children especially in their teens often gets disrespectful and violent towards their loved one.They have these thoughts that entire World is nice and only their parents are their enemies! Would you like to join me for a Pop concert tonight for a change? Martin's are in the city i told him and in no time his mood changed.Martin's were his favourite,i drove him to the concert. We had a hearty meal and his favourite Havmor ice cream on the way back ! I'll talk to you tomorrow Nisha i said her as i dropped him back home.

Next day at 11am she knocked my OPD door and sat in front of me.What did he say? She asked me frowning. You are finding Neverlands Nisha i told her. What?? She screamed in dismay.Yeah you are trying to find lands where you have never been,you and Amit couldn't crack civil exams and you both want rishab to crack it, you have made his life nothing but a timetable. Whatever you couldn't do or achieve in your lives you want him to do that not for him but basically for you. You guys are overburdening him with your expectations.He is no doubt a brilliant guy but your constant comparison, constant instructions is making him tensed. You are trying finding Neverlands but this land does not even exist for him. It's called FOMO..fear of missing out. He is getting depressed by thinking if he won't live upto your expectations he will be out of your good wills and if he won't mingle with his friends he will be thrown out of his peer circles this constant stress and fear is making him equally violent and silent.It's called Maniac depressive disorder where people sometimes are too hyper and often gets violent in Maniac phase and later they get too depressed and goes into shell cutting off everything with outer world.

Now what should I do?Nisha was scared by this now, she never imagined her Son might be undergoing so much stress and emotional turmoil. Set him free...let him do what he likes...he is good at cricket...let him enjoy it with his friends. Let him party for a while and go for movies sometimes.Everyone needs break yaar...i told her. Don't be too strict and harsh on him you can see his falling grades in last few semesters. You never heard him Nisha. Amit and you always were busy earning to give him best life but you both missed best time in your life with your child. Most important thing in child's growing period is to be with him,to hear him. Parents should be his best friends where he can share everything...try to be his cool friends than parents and you will see the change in him. I prescribed some tablets for him,she understood the therapy needed and she left.

Few months later Nisha called me. Rishab won Man of the Match in the District cricket tournament she was telling happily. Ohh that's great but how did this all happened i asked. After i left your clinic i went to Amit's office and discussed what you had told me. We realised our mistakes.From the next day we stopped being over protective and over reactive parents, we let him sleep till late somedays, we encouraged him to go for cricket practice.We called his friends home for party and even booked their tickets for the movie. After few days we could see changes in Rishabh. He looked more relaxed and his mood was more stabilised with your medication too. He started opening up to us. We started spending all our time at home with him and started having dinner together. Few days after enjoyment he started realising his responsibilities by himself and he started studying well. We both are very happy for him. Next month we have booked him Dubai trip,he wanted to have world's largest and tallest ride at Safari world she was chirping continuously. I was happy my therapy worked both medicines and counseling.Teer sahi nishane pe laga tha. After all she is a mother and mother can never go wrong for her child...i smiled!

* * *

CHAPTER 8

MODERN MONALISAS

Our lives are the stories in which we write, direct and star in the leading role.Some scenes are happy while others bring lessons to learn but we have the power to be the heros of our own adventure.After all who doesnt like to be the star in the lead? Influenced by the flawless beauty of Deepika in Pathaan and Genelia in Ved, i too got tempted to pamper myself and then instantly booked my appointment in my regular saloon.As i was climbing the stairs and entering the saloon i met these Modern Monalisas- Wonder Women of today's generation.

These were two young and beautiful girls on the wheel chairs getting their hair spa done.I was bit taken aback and shocked to see this scenario as this was something very new to me.Have never seen such disabled ladies enjoying spa sessions and parlour services relaxingly.They were wheel chair bound and they had no sensations below their waist.Their legs were numb and they couldn't walk.Their wheel chair being their best friend but their condition did not deter their inner strength and they looked soo strong and bright.

Waiting for my turn and sitting on the reclining sofa in the saloon lobby and Starring at them my doctor mind was busy analysing their condition trying to reach the diagnosis.Paraplegia?Spinal injuries? Myopathies? Muscular dysthropy?? What it could be? My curious mind started working.What happened to them? I just poked my question silently to the girl and the man sitting next to me assuming them to be their relatives.They both have Friedrich's Ataxia he mumbled slowly and it moved the ground beneath me. What..? Friedrich's Ataxia? I almost screamed.It was the last thing anybody would want for them.

Friedrich's Ataxia is a genetic disorder in which person looses his sensation in the legs, the trunk become weak,legs looses it's power and strength.It progress gradually and after first decade of life they are wheel chair bound.The condition keeps worsening with the age,shortening their life span and as it is genetic it can be passed on to the next generations.The name of this disease shattered me from within and here were these two young beautiful warriors fighting their lives with great Elan!!

Are you related to them? I asked the lady sitting next to me.Yeah they are my sister's.I'm the youngest and this is my husband,she introduced the robust man with long hair in a pony tail to me.We just got married a week ago she updated.And here they were together accompanying her wheel chair bound sisters to the saloon.This was something very new, very unique to me!!

They both finished their services and these two now went to get things done. Both those girls pressed the start button of their electric wheelchair and came next to me. I gave them a familiar smile. Yeah within some time i had got to know them and their story.So what do you do?still studying? I asked them curiously. Nooo... they gave a big smile.We both are working.I work for German MNC and she works for Japanese company. I was flabbergasted by their input.You both work ? I asked with a wide face.Yes they said calmly. We went to school on a wheelchair, played rugby.We even played wheelchair dandiya in our school gatherings, participated in lemon on spoon game sitting on the wheelchair and even won it.We even cook our food and roll our rotis being on this chair.We are the Disney Princess and hence are offered this special seats...they giggled in happiness.

I was awe struck with their reactions.There was no sadness,there was no grief, no question of why me? no anxiety of what's next? They have very well understood that life is not a problem to be solved but a reality to be expirenced and accepted.Both of them were living their life to the fullest and with grace. But it's not easy to digest the fact that two daughters of the same family are affected with such a crippling disease and are dependent on wheelchair in such a young age.But kudos to their parents and siblings who were always motivating them and supporting them to be the best version of themselves. In any unfavorable circumstances we have two choices one to sit and crib blaming our fate or to rise and fight against the situation and overcome the tide.And no doubt these two sisters have choosen the second option showing the world that nothing is impossible, the word itself says I'm possible!

So Enjoying life haa...i asked them with a smile. And they said yess...Mam we know we are born with this and even if we want we can't change it. We have accepted our lives this way and try to make the best out of it.We know our lives are short and hence we want to make every moment of this journey memorable so when we are gone we will be still here with our loved ones with these eternal memories.

We go to the Spa, we pamper ourselves in the saloon,we go for shopping.We go on to the trips,we even went to Himalayan excursions...they were telling excitedly.Someday we all have to go..so why not dare to live? Their talks were amazingly inspirational like their lives.Till that time a guy came with many ice cream cones packed neatly.He started distributing those ice creams to everyone in the saloon.They smiled at me and said take Mam,it's from us to all these lovely people here who help us feel relaxed and look beautiful with their amazing parlour services.They removed their phones and started making insta reel showing their double layered ice cream cones." Yeh hum hai and yeh humari sister and brother in law hai, hum spa karwa re hai and humari Pawri hori hai!" Their stylish look and melodious voice added more beauty to their insta reel. I was really stunned with their courage to fight the Life's every odd!

Their sister and brother in law finished their services and came to us.Ok madam will leave now her sister said. It's nice meeting you .Both my sister's are looking soo happy talking to you.We stay nearby so visit us sometimes when you get time.I nodded my head with a smile. They started their electrical chair and moved one after another and waited near the stairs. Their brother in law and one more person from the saloon lifted their chair and took them to the car.He lifted them in his arms one by one and put them into the rear seat and assured if they were comfortable.Both of them were looking out of the window and waving happily at me. Their shinny spa hair and happy glowing faces were making them more radiant. I kept seeing them till their car went far out of my sight.

Truly these two girls felt like Modern Monalisas to me. Life has thrown lemons to them and they were enjoying the lemonade out of it.They were the stone of hope from the Mountain of despair. I appreciated their will power and the way they have defined their own lives.Instead of crying over their disability they choose to trust the journey and embrace the life.They were like those strong walls which shakes but never collapse.The unity and solidarity among these three sisters moved my heart and the generosity of their brother in law and his quality to accept them with big heart touched my soul.Their story is a big lesson to those all who gets depressed and frustrated with their small failures.When these wheel chair bound disable girls can go to parlour, get hair spa, can dine out in the restaurant,can go for shopping and even can do the jobs why the other people often gets upset with the minor things going wrong in their life.These two girls showed us success is not final, failure is not fatal but it's the courage to continue that is what counts.Finally it's not how long we live but how well we live is all that matters.And hence these two wheel chair bound girls are the real stars of their lives who scripted their own story and made it a Blockbuster....!! Really some people are truly Miraculous and some stories are truly Magical....Just like this one!!

* * *

CHAPTER 9
75 & NOT OUT

In the life of our's we come across many people,meet different characters, people with different nature,differnt culture,people with different mentality. Some real,some fake,some helpful,some acting to be helpful. Some one genuine and some gem of the people.Some we forget over a time period but few make permenant mark on you. I always say my profession shows me rainbow of emotions and i live hundreds of life in one! Working in the pediatric setup with young kids i was quiet fortunate to meet this young man who was mere 75 years old. Yeah just 75 years and counting! And he made me believe that age is just a number! I have seen people who gets older and weared out in their 40's. Morely mental ageing than physical whereas seeing this young gentleman of 75 years made me realise only your body ages and not your soul!

I was sitting on a bench in the front yard park of an extremely busy orthopedic hospital seeing varieties of people crossing across the road.They were of different ages,different religions,different problems, someones hand in plaster,someone operated with hip joints,some had underwent knee operations some rehabilitating from RTA's.Among the crowd came ahead a grandpa tall,sturdily built with big white moustache, White kurta and White dhoti on but his face was glowing white with his pain and agonies leaving behind.A broad big smile lightened his face as he approached me slowly holding his walker tight.You are Dr wali's daughter? A very familiar question to me still in the area of my hometown where I am still being known as Dr Wali's daughter despite today i being the most accomplished person in self with very much of my own independent identity at my work place.Still i feel proud to be called as Dr Wali's daughter as it tickles that little girly in me who is always been proud of being daddy's little girl courtesy my dad's aura and fame!! Yes i said softly. I'm Mr Patil,you don't know me but i have seen you and your sister closely since your childhood.

We used to regularly visit your Dad as his patient.It was again a regular introduction as most of the people from my hometown are my Dad's patients. I gave him that familiar smile of "ohhh is it.??.He sat beside me on the bench and said "Donhi gudghyacha operation karun ghetaloya." in that typical kannada mixed marathi accent popularly known as border language.I smiled heartily as i heard this kannada marathi mix slang after quiet a lot time.You know what this is my 5th operation in the last 5 years,average one per year haa...haa..haa came out the loud laugh behind his face wincing with pain travelling down his legs.Heart surgery - bypass in 2014, kindney operation for stones in 2015,Cataract operation in both eyes in 2016 and 2017 and now Knee replacement both sides in 2018 getting new body parts installed yearly one making me younger and healthier haa..haa..ha....laughter reaching the clouds followed.I knew the pain was much bigger than his big loud laugh.Undergoing major surgeries that too every year spending hell lot of time in various hospitals and that too with such a positive attitude requires lots of courage and who else will know it better than a doctor itself?.

I see lots of patients going through mental,physical and financial trauma daily day in-out & counselling these patients on these very aspect being part of my profession.

Do you have severe pain Ajoba? I asked him looking at his painful face.Not at all young girl pailwans don't feel this small pains.You know i'm state level wrestler of my time.Have won many kustis on this khasbaugh maidan, famous land of wrestling in kolhapur."Sagli Ambabaichi krupa"but that wrestling fights took toll on my joints orelse my knees would have been stronger till i beat my century. His sense of humour was great! You know i used to drink 6 litres of milk daily and used to do 1300 of sit ups daily, i was just shocked and felt as if i got atrial fibrillations..13;00 not at all a joke!

He slowly removed a big paper from his pocket and handed it to me.I curiously opened it and found a beautiful sketch of Dr Vaidya a well known chief operating orthopaedic surgeon with a world record who has operated on him as well.You have sketched it?One more surprise came from behind.Yeah said the old young man with his familiar smile.I have done lots of beautiful paintings right from Shivaji Maharaj to Swami Vivekanand to Abdul Kalam.I just see some picture or person for a while and then draw them spontaneously.I generally take 2 and a half hour to sketch one.Come sometimes home and you can see my sketches he said warmly.What a brilliant sketch he has made of Dr Vaidya,more original than real with same glowy eyes full of confidence.I had brought this to gift him as a token of my gratitude towards him for making me walk again on my both legs he added humbly. I was just statue still with back to back surprises he threw at me. I was totally unprepared for this one!

I have made huge live size photo sketch of Sri Swami Samartha of Akkalkot,i'm huge devotee of Swami Samartha and have built his temple near my house in my farm.

" Bhivu Nakos; mi tuzya pathishi aahe".I'm living my entire

life fearlessly on this sentence of swami.Whenever i'm in pain,in anger,in disguise,in despair when i'm lost and feel defeated i just sit in front of his idol in this my temple to pray wholeheartedly and you know what my all troubles gets lighter instantly.Swami guides my life he told me his secret. I realised instantly from where his all energy,courage and positivity comes from.It's from his heavenly abode and his deep trust in his Swami Samarth.

It was getting darker.Sun has set long back,his golden rays had turned mauve and fiery red to get immeresed in the blue sky. Moon was trying to peep from behind the clouds making it more serene."Katarvel"we call it in marathi where deep silence speak volumes in the nature.A sense of hollowness,sense of unknown insecurity dives within us.

"Chaand milta nahi har kisiko;yeh diye ki roshni kya kam hain humko" ? he said emotionally ,his voice trembled.Oh grandpaa you do poems as well? That too hindi at this age? I was litreally blown by this time. It was just unbelivable.Yeah i'm a voracious reader. I have hundreds of Marathi and Hindi poetry books of all the renowned poets in my personal library and you will always find 2- 3 poetry books lying besides my pillow.I read them before i sleep, my new lenses in my eyes makes the letters more brighter now. The same smile flashed again" Jinko mana apna sab kuch,unn logo ne hi mara khanjir pithapar...Par yeh buland hosale kya kam hain; apni zindagi bithane haskar"one more meaningful lines from his poem.It was too deep,emotional yet powerful.He got up and started walking struggling with his walker trying to hide the tears rolling down his cheeks."Ayengi mushkilye anek zindagi mein; datkar samna karna; ek mila tha shaksh aisa bhi ,bus.. duaon mein yaad rakhna" he mumbled as he walked.I just kept looking at his image going far and far in the moonlight making the atmosphere more darker.Truly these old people bring true light and courage to enlighten our younger generation who often falls prey to depression by slightest things going wrong in our life." Pata nahi kahan se aati hain inn mei itni himmat". I was just thinking to myself when my Dad came searching for me.Ohh you are here...i was looking for you everywhere.By the way what are you doing here? I came out of my thoughts and said with a smile"Kahi nahi dad; mala ek avaliya bhetala".Chand milta nahi har kisiko,yeh diye ki roshni bhi kya kam hain humko! To be happy and content with the life we have got- is the key!! And i started walking with my Dad.I could feel the moon smiling from above showering his cool beams on me!!! 75 and not out...and still a dark horse... amazingly versatile! A real Avaliya!! Really sometimes miracles come in a bundle...like this one!!!

* * *

CHAPTER 10
A TALE OF TWO STATES

Sitting in the friday OPD surrounded by the maddening crowd i was busy checking our VLBW (very low birth weight babies) babies who had come for the follow up's after their discharge." High risk follow up OPD" is what we call it as and its one of the busiest day of the week.69 from the morning and still counting...i just dialled the reception number with all my strength “One coffee for me veronica" i ordered a cup of hot coffee for me to rejuvenate myself to pull the next crowd coming.A gentle knock on my opd door,yes please come in i whispered with whatever little energy i had. I could see one bouquet of flowers coming almost flying in my room.I was bit shocked and kept my eyes wide open but couldn't see anyone.Till that time almost that bouquet had reached my table and then swiped a beautiful chubby face behind those refreshing flowers.

Who are you? I asked amusingly as he looked too big for our follow up opd. I'm Anshuman,he came out from behind the bouquet and flashed his warm smile. I have come to meet you,i just passed my 1st std and have excelled in my exam and he put a box full of sweets in front of me.This too is for you he said warmly.Till now i was trying to figure out who he was.Looking at my confused face he repeated again,im Anshuman from Dibrugarh Assam.Now suddenly my brain got recharged.Ohhh yes..Anshuman....i could recall his cubby face,small eyes while we shifted him to our Nicu in a small transport trolley.His parents were standing worried in our counselling room with heaps of papers,medical documents which they carried from Dibrugarh hospital.We shifted him in our warmer.One and a half month old baby still weighing only 3 kgs.He looked sick,pale with huge abdomen,most of his weight was due to his swollen abdomen.Multiple small rashes over his limbs.His breathing was fast and acidotic.Baby was almost gasping.I immediately intubated and connected him to the ventilator.Now machine was taking care of his breathing and he was on artificial respiration.He was septic and in shock.We drew his blood samples and started him on the treatment with iv fluids,BP controlling medicines,antibiotics and other supportive measures as he got stabilised on the ventilator.I walked to my counselling room to talk to his attenders.

Hello I'm your baby's doctor, newborn specialist.Yes doctor we have travelled all the way from Assam.This is our only son born after 18 years of our marriage.Mother is elderly so she didnt had enough breast milk so we fed him with the cow's milk and formula milk.And now he started having this problem of abdominal fullness,stomach bloating up and he has become dull, not accepting feeds.Doctors at Assam told us he requires human milk and we have been transferred here as you have human milk bank in your unit. Parents told their story. Yeah your baby is suffering from cow's milk protein intolerance.He is not able to digest the cow's milk.His intestines are swollen up because of infection. He is critically ill on ventilatory support but you have to be strong and patient. We will try our level best i assured the parents.

These were elite rich parents well read and well educated who came all the way long from Assam for the treatment of their only son who was indeed a precious child born after 18 years.Naturally parents looked bit old. Reports came in and i was shocked as his Hb was 6 gms and platelets read as only 4000 against 1.5 lakhs as normal count. We pumped him with the higher antibiotics,platelet transfusion, blood transfusion and FFP. We gambled with almost all the available drugs to control his infection.We spent hours together under the laminar flow to prepare his special i.v nutrition i.e TPN calculating his daily calorie and protein requirements.The parents had booked a hotel room next to our hospital and spent months together praying and treating their child.Their extended family of aunts who were on the top official position being High court judge,Revenue officers and so on joined their parents to help them out. Money was not an issue for them but patience was.We were literally playing a war with his infection without any much bright picutre with only hope that some day we could see his platelets improving.

No doubt we have pumped him n numbers of platelets,plasma and blood transfusions to keep him alive. Months passed by and God answered our hard work and parents prayers.Baby started showing some improvement.Abdomen fullness decreased and became soft,his color improved and breathing normalised.We prayed to god for his safe extubation i.e safe removal of his airway tube which we have put in to maintain his breathing.This was the third intubation for the baby in 2 months of his hospital stay.In these two months i realised what its to be blank,to be square,to be puzzled and so on.As we were just treating and treating putting all my medical knowldge to stake but unsure of his outcome.Now he was 3 and half months and i really felt kudos for the patience and perseverance of their parents who just had immense faith in our treatment and never questioned nor doubted a single thing.Their rock steady belief in us doubled our confidence.We started feeding him slowly with the human milk from our milk bank.Indeed human milk was liquid gold for this baby. It was the time when elementary formulas were not availble

freely so only hope to save this child was human milk which was screened for infections and stored hygenically in specialised deep freeze unit calld as Milk Bank. The mothers who had excess milk post delivery donated their milk to these banks where it is processed and stored safely and utilised for the babies in need. I was lucky enough to work in the unit where we had this facility as very few harldly 5-6 centres in entire india had this facility of milk banking we being one of them.!! He drank gallons and gallons of milk in next 1 month from our milk bank and was ready with his new look.He gained weight,had healthy glow.His face became cheerful and so of his parents. His infection was totally controlled. His tummy was soft as he digested human milk properly and gained adequate weight. His stay was the longest in our unit of full 3 months. At the time of discharge he looked like a young handsome lad.

Their parents couldn't stop praising us and we were overwhelmed with their gratitude.They distributed sweets in the entire hospital and i couldn't forget his sparkling eyes.He was nursed by 2 wet nurses at guwahati who fed him their milk till age of 6 months after which he was weaned to the normal diet.They kept sending his pictures of growing up to me and our nicu sisters on and off. And today he was here in front of me standing tall and sturdy with his refreshing smile like those of refreshing flowers in the bouquet.I could not belive a small sick lifeless bacchu lying listless in our nicu bed to grow up into this handsome lad today. His journey was stormy indeed and i was stunned to recall how many multiples of transfusions we have given to keep him alive. His sparkling eyes sparkled more as his words kept resounding in my ears I'm Anshuman from

Assam.His parents followed with a big cake inside my room.Today is his 6th birthday mam and we want to cherish this moment with you who gave him this new life.We are forever grateful to you.Tears rolled down their cheeks. Tears of joy,happiness and gladness all mixed in one." Happiest birthday Anshuman....Live long long life" i wished him dearly. I thanked god for choosing me to treat these kids and help them live new life. No doubt the cake tasted more sweet. Moment of perfect blend of happiness and satisfaction. Moment which sealed the union of two states and many lives......Indeed a kodak moment to cherish life long!!!!

P.S.: Cow's milk protein intolerance (CMPI) is a deadly and serious life threatening illness seen in the babies fed with cows milk. Proteins in the cow's milk are heavy to digest for the newborns and can cause necrotising enterocolitis i.e severe infection of the intestines leading to multi organ dysfunction. So do not feed your newborn babies with cow's,buffalo,goat or any other milk diluted or undiluted. Mother's milk is the best milk for her child.It's the Liquid Gold for the babies.If not available feed the babies with appropriate milk formulas with your doctors advice.Healthy babies makes Healthy nation!!

* * *

CHAPTER 11

THE GOOD FELLA

Go straight and then right.....Lady receptionist smiled and instructed me. I collected my room keys and walked through the beautiful campus of the most renowned children hospital of Banglore.It was month of july and cold waves and mansoon showers were hitting everywhere. It was chilled outside but pleasant.Green trees were stand still as they were frozen in this freezing cold.Clouds were flying high making the sky blur and the sun was also getting lazy to rise in this rains.Won't his mother be scolding him if he gets up so late? Like our mom's scold us? I thought to myself and laughed on my own silly notion!

I reached my room 107, alloted to me on the ground floor.As i was opening the door i saw a young lad of 8-9 years peeping out of his room curiously.Chubby cheeks, big eyes and with the bigger smile he looked naughty. Before i could say anything he jumped inside his room and disappeared.For the next two months this room was my home as i was posted for my peripheral postings here at India's famous Children and Cancer hospital.The room was neat and tidy.Big window made it more airy and lit.I always loved well ventilated rooms.A table was on the right side with sturdy wooden chair and table lamp on it,left side was the bed with clean bedsheet spread on it and a pillow and blanket neatly placed.Inbuilt cupboards were there in walls to keep my luggage,clothes and books.I went into the bathroom, splashed cold water on my face and felt refreshed.As i came out i saw the same neighbouring boy standing in my room.Hey hi....what's your name? i asked him. I'm Ganesha he told boldly.So you are going to stay here from today? Which department? he asked as he continued to wander in my room touching all the things i have just spread on the table and continuously pressing on and off button of the table lamp.

Pediatrics i told him my department name obidently.He waited for a moment and saw me again "but you are too big to be treated there" he said confusingly.ohhh i started laughing...no.. no.. no...I'm not here for treatment,I'm a doctor who came here to treat these sick children and learn,I'm posted here for my studies i tried explaining to him in the most simple language that i can.Ohhh then why you staying here? All the doctors stay on the first floor of this building...this is patients floor he said impatiently.Yeah I know but upstairs all rooms are full so i got alloted this room i told him. Now he got my point why I was here with the books and all.Where is the canteen here? i need some tea i asked him.Ohhh tea...come I'll take you he swinged front and back of me as I walked through the corridor.

He accompanied me to the canteen. I sat on the chair, waiting for the Stuart to come and take my order,"Le Rajanna, baro ille, hosa madam bandidare...tinde Kodi aulage";he informed him loudly in kannada.What you will have madam?Rajanna asked me politely.Idly,wada, poori,upma, dosa, sheera, Pongal?? Idly teeni madam superr ga irrathe ili....Ganesha informed me to have idlis there as those very supersoft and tasty.After having idly and coffee i came back to my room to rest and Ganesha went to his room informing me he will come back again later. If you need something tell me madam he said while leaving and he jumped into his room.

This was totally a new place for me and i knew nothing.Ganesha helped me to book my meals daily with Gouramma who used to supply food boxes daily to all the doctors here.He showed me the departmental stores nearby where we get our daily essentials,he showed me the bakery and good restaurants nearby.He pointed to a small gate on the opposite side of the road.."that is Nimhans campus madam.It's too good and huge,lots of trees and greenery inside,you can go there for your morning walk. Many people do jogging there" he gave me another input.So in short he was my local guide there at IGICH.Whenever i needed something this little kid used to come along and keep advising me and informing me about everything within the campus and outside too.He was my local Google!

He often arrived at my room uninformed and kept continuously ranting about everything under the sky.He was very intelligent and impatient,always busy touching things, throwing something, wandering here there.His mother too started making short trips to my room along with him.They belonged to a small village from deep Karnataka and were staying here for his treatment.He was suffering from leukemia (blood cancer) and was undergoing chemotherapy.So many blood tests, scans and chemotherapy for such a small child still he was so happy and living his life to the fullest.Every year they used to visit IGICH multiple times and stay here for 2-3 months.Some time he used to get high grade fever because of very low WBC counts, loose motions, frequent infections,gastritis due to medicines,his hair were getting sparse and so his mother had cut all his hair. His shiny head brought much shine to his face,his legs used to pain but still he was never tierd of jumping and mocking around.Life was slowing for him but he never slowed down.With deep pains and aches he kept his smile alive.He knew each and every person in that hospital very well,it was like his second home.

All the Doctors were his friends,they used to call him while climbing up or down the stairs.Nange chocolate tarlilva?He used to ask them if they haven't bought him chocolates and they used to advise him to eat good fruits.In the evening he used to play in the small park in front of our rooms. He used to pick up frogs near the pond and used to run behind other kids scaring them.Once they all are gone and hidden into their rooms he used to see at frog and used to laugh out loud I'll eat you now,he used to tell the struggling frog trying to get out of his hands and dip into the pond. Biddo maharaya, ninge bere kelsa ilva Ganesha? Shankar watchman used to scold him in kannada for harassing the frog then he used to dip that frog back in the pond and run to his room.

Every night some strange sounds used to come from my room, sometimes from cupboard and sometimes beneath my bed.I used to get up in the middle of night and keep searching who was making that sound putting on all the lights but no one was seen.I used to drench in sweat as i have heard some ghost stories here in this campus.Next day Ganesha came as usual to my room and i gently told about the strange noises coming out of my room at night and asked him if he knew something about the ghosts here.Ghost? he started laughing.I will do arrangements of all those ghosts madam he said and left.After some times he came with wooden planks, hammer and some nails and started fixing it on the lower side of my door.What you doing?? I asked him confusingly.I'm fixing the entry of the ghost in your room madam he said funnily and after much hardwork of more than a hour he fixed that wooden plank to my door.And to my disbelief those sounds stopped coming from that night.I asked him what did he do? He took me out to the small park just outside the rooms that evening and i could see many rats playing, running one after another.Ohh my God...i screamed.These are your ghosts madam,night they enter our rooms from the gap below the door and keep making sounds he informed.I was relived to know the mystery behind those loud noise and strange sounds in my room and slept peacefully that night.

I enquired about Ganesha's illness with my colleagues over there.It's stage 4 leukemia with widespread secondaries and Metastasis all over his body.He won't be surviving more than a month or two they informed me.I felt shattered and i was thrown down in the deep valley of sorrows and grief.Looking at my worried and depressed face in the evening he got to know what i was thinking.So you got to know about me?he asked calmly.Yeah are you aware about your illness? Yes mam I'm having stage 4 leukemia with widespread metastasis and wouldn't be living for more than a month..that's what your friends have told you right?he said Coldly. I was shocked he knew everything but still he was soo calm and composed. Mam your friends are foolish, they don't know even bit of their subject, see how fit I'm.I ask them to get chocolates for me and they tell me to eat fruits instead.They want to send me for Yamraj visit sooner but don't worry mam i know their tricks so i won't eat fruits and won't go to yamraj earlier he started smiling.I took out dairy milk from my bag and gave it to him,he disappeared in the dark. Knowing everything about his illness and having few days to count in his life still he was soo strong and was dealing his battle courageously.

From where these kids gets this power??Two months were over and then i moved out of IGICH hospital premises and went on with my course.I was busy with my new patients but i always remembered Ganesha.He was always in my thoughts and prayers.One afternoon as i was bit relaxing after my lunch our ward boy came with a letter, it's for you mam he handed over to me. I opened it curiously.It was a very shabbily written letter, handwriting was not clear, letters were ups and down...it was from Ganesha." Mam I feel today is my last day,after this I'll be going forever. I always remember you.502 is the number of maintenance department, call them if you need some repair i won't be there with you now on to help you"...i read the letter with heavy heart. Tears started rolling down my cheeks profusely.Some lives touch our heart so deeply.

I called on his mother's number, Anju can i speak to Ganesha? i asked her and she started sobbing badly. Ganesha left us four days back madam..he was very sick and breathless.He was remembering you often and insisted he will write you a letter himself.He was not in the position to sit up in the bed still he managed to write 2-3 lines for you somehow.. she started weeping.I felt sudden hollowness in my stomach, a sense of insecurity surrounded me. Who will accompany me to the canteen, morning walks, hospital wards and to the garden ponds? who will scare me with green yellow frogs and who will throw the ghosts out of my room?who will tell me romcom stories of nurses link-up to wardboys and other people?my saviour has gone forever...i felt like i was suddenly an orphan.I saw out of my window... it was dark and cloudy,it was raining heavily both outside and inside me too.Suddenly a lightening flashed my window followed by a thunder.What have you dropped now Ganesha there in the sky? I screamed looking out of the window towards the sky above.I knew he was there in a better and safe place now for sure! This Good fella was in God's hand now!!

* * *

CHAPTER 12
PLANET HUMANITY

As a child i always heard that there are 8 planets in the galaxy and i just got to know the 9th one. Just like the 9th wonder of the world,the 9th planet.Planet humanity,yes just like the moon, the stars and the other planets revolve around the sun creating the cosmic connections human emotions and notions revolves around each other creating some really great cosmic and divine connection as i realised this one!

Triage alarm beeped as it signaled the new case arrival in the triage room. I marched towards the triage OPD to receive the case just to find our foundation worker carrying a very small fragile baby wrapped in a worned out torn cotton saree piece.As he placed the small one on the warmer bed his weak cry and feeble movements showed his sign of life. This one is from chinchu tanda,born 10 days back.They were feeding him milk drops with a leaf.We traced them and got him here foundation worker briefed us about the case.I instructed my PG's for the further treatment.Sugars were low,baby was IUGR and morsoever severely dehydrated throwing multiple apneas.We put the baby on the ventilator,started all the needed treatment and after settling the baby i turned towards the attenders to give them the update.These were the Chinchus,a well known tribal community of Telagana located in a deep foresty areas.A man in the 30's in typical tribal attire followed by a young lady in early 20's

(or in teenage?) accompanied by an old lady in typical tribal wear with half worn saree till knee length without blouse,a big nose ring swagging down and hands full of ivory white big bangles entered the room.This scene was quite common for me as i worked at this hospital which was attached to the foundation.These foundation workers are catered to deep hilly and forest areas which are literally unreachable.They travel through the rivers and water canals in the small boats to reach these tandas,find out pregnant ladies and the newborn babies in the need of the treatment and shift to our hospital for the special care.Looking at their commendable job i always refer them as the angels of today's era! I counselled parents regarding the baby's condition and told our foundation worker to make their staying arrangements in the wing specially made for rural folk.They followed him with morose look albiet reluctantly.

We placed this baby in the premature ward next to the baby of almost similar weight.This baby was one of the twins.Parents of the twin babies were highly educated couple owning a pharma company who had tried almost all the possible routes for conceiving the baby but had failed several times.And now using ivf conception could become proud parents of twin babies.These babies too were premature both weighing 1 kg and 1.2 kgs.One twin had died few days back due to multiple problems of prematurity and from that day this other twin had also stopped showing signs of improvement.We started treating both these primis with great care. I could see the picture of two worlds both poles apart.One baby from the 1st world country born to the educated rich parents and other one from the 3rd world country born to uneducated parents.Two worlds together at the same time same moment.Rich or poor,educated or illiterate,hitech or laid back....agonies are distributed equally for all! Our job was to treat them both with immense devotion to make them well.Treatment was going on and both little fighters were trying to change their games.Both were off ventilator and on full feeds.We involved both mothers in feeding.Educated mother looked worried and was trying hard to feed her little one with paladay taking care of all the possible hygiene and asepsis.Most of the baby care products were brought from the USA and other side was this young Chinchu woman looking fully confused and depressed and trying to feed her baby unwillingly with zero intrest.

Next day i called all the attenders for counselling only to find that our Chinchu mother was absconding and had ran away from the hospital.Her husband and mother in law stood looking helpless in front of me getting fired from our foundation worker in their tribal language.She couldn't adjust to this city life madam,her husband tried telling me.It wasn't a new thing for me at all as these tribals are not used to the city life style.I could sense that uneasiness in their behaviour. They could not sit on the dining table in the hospital canteen and eat food.They couldn't sleep on the bed. They are not used to be among these suit boot modern people.They are the rustic people used to earthy lifestyle.Eating raw food and sleeping under the open sky.They are wild wanderers in the green jungles and not meant to be in this cement jungle.I laughed at myself thinking how foolish i was to teach them hand washing and basics of sanitation without knowing their ground reality.Where are they going to follow this six steps of handwashing in their hills and from which tree are they going to procure sanitizers? We should be realistic and rationale while treating our patients.These people taught me to think!

Okay...you too go to your tanda, discuss with the baby's mother and convince her to get back here to nurse your baby.Meanwhile our nurses (i fondly call them foster mothers)will take care of your baby I told the baby's father and granny.Treatment was going on but our hearts shattered as we found out that this baby had a large hole in the septum of heart (perimembranous VSD) which would require surgery in the later life.After few days our foundation workers got the mother back to the hospital.She was reluctant to take the baby and looked depressed.I don't want this baby,i already have two babies at home and again in a year or so i can have another one she said bluntly.What will i do with this baby with a heart problem? But it's treatable and foundation will help you for the surgery i told her. No i don't want to stay here,she started crying.And almost threatening her husband in her language to take her back.Okay madam will take our baby they told us.What will you do with him? i asked them worriedly. In our community if babies have defects we think that God has not made them eligible to survive in this world.We keep them on the bush and leave them on their own fate he told mi without any emotion.Whattttttt i almost screamed.This is totally inhuman.i can't allow you to do that.You don't want this baby it's okay, we will take care. And thus baby went to Nicu under the foundation care and parents back to their tribe. I spent many sleepless nights thinking about all these facts,i don't know what is right and what is wrong but yes still these things exist even in today's world.

May i come in mam? soft voice broke my thoughts. I saw educated parents of twin baby entering my room. Mam we want to adopt that small baby.We know the history and we have made our mind to take care of him. We have observed the day this baby came into the next warmer of our baby,his voice,cry,movements have put life in our baby. It was where this baby's other twin was kept.Our baby started improving and tolerating feeds in this baby's company.We will operate on him and treat him as our other twin child they spoke warmly but firmly. A sense of relief spread on my face. I thought for a while,Ok if your decision is final I'll talk to our management for legal adoption i told them assuringly.This baby will get a family and they will get their twins.What could be more delightful and blissful. I went to the Nicu and saw two primie warriors sleeping peacefully in the two neighbouring warmers.Twinny buddies they are...i said to myself.A million dollar smile flashed on my face.And i thought there are many many planets in the galaxy....Urban planet,rural planet,illiterate planet and a modern planet,Green planet,Cement planet but biggest planet is PLANET HUMANITY!And then there are these cosmic rays emerging from this planet and connecting all other planets in one galaxy!! Yes humanity still do exist and some miracles are seen like this!!

* * *

CHAPTER 13
DIE HEALTHY

The hall was full house. Everyone was ready in their clean clothes sitting on their respective yoga mats. It was the time to start the programme by now but i was impatiently waiting for one person. My eyes twinkled as I saw her coming.She slowly walked in her properly organised 9 yard kasota Saree with a white bun of little hair tied on her crown. Her face had that bright shine and glow. She was 87 years but still had that child like energy and charm of 16 years old girl.She went to her regular place,spread her yoga mat, sat with her back straight with folding hands. And now i started Aum with a broad smile. It was an International Yoga day and we have organised the yoga programme at my place. Since couple of years the yoga craze and trend has seen a steep rise in India and abroad.Our ancient yoga has travelled worldwide.In my childhood I did basic yoga class and i found it quiet boring and disinteresting.

Moreover to rise early before the sun rise and taking yoga mat and walking to yoga class in half asleep mode was too cumbersome for me in those early days. But time changes and so as we. As i grew I started understanding the core importance of yoga.

The science behind the Asanas and being into the most strenuous and stressful job of ICU I slowly started valuing mental peace a lot over everything else and my inclination towards this ancient indian art grew many folds. I always believe sharing is caring. And i do share every small and big information of public use to one and all who are in my regular touch. People associated with me always enjoy my intellectual talks and they always feel their GK improves leaps and bounds after hearing to my talks on each and every matter under this sky.Yes i can talk about politics,international affairs,cricket,bollywood, human rights, education system and their flaws and off course on human relationships too. I have always been vocal and opinionated with strong leadership quality and hence people always believed me firmly and my ideas strongly and so i too strive hard to make it a reality. And this Yoga awareness class too was one of my brainchild.

So shall we start 6am yoga club? I just initiated this topic over the cup of hot piping tea after our daily ward rounds. My team mates just splurged their tea and looked at me with that sarcastic look.Who will join? And where to start? They asked in a disintrested way. Yeah they may have thought i got this impulse from various pictures of celebrities in the different yoga poses trending on social media and advertisements in the newspapers. Do you want to get clicked for yoga day and pose in different Aasanas and put it on FB or Whats app status? If that's so let's go to some hilly areas or green terrain, click some pictures and come back.That way we will have one day trip in nature's lap and your job of clicking pictures also will be done..they mocked me smiling.

No.. I'm not a social media fringy to put pictures for showcasing i said in a serious tone. By this time they knew some ideas were deep rooting in my brain and my neurons will produce something extra ordinary in the short time. What's you are upto? They asked curiously. We will have 20 mins yoga session daily in our hospital before we start our day at work.We will involve all our staff and patients too so that they could get awareness and intrest in this field.As a doctor our goal should not be treating illness but rather transforming ourselves into our improvised healthy version so as to keep the diseases at the bay! I was talking in a flow. So we need not wake up early and come to your 6am club they said cheekily after hearing me completly and carefully. Let's start with this short session first and let's see how it goes. And that's how we started with our brief yoga sessions which were so much fun. Less time but more enjoyable and not even boring too. Everyone started feeling healthy vibes and almost everyone were looking forward for next day session.

Slowly I started my 6 am club too and it was open for everyone. I found space in our car garage which was huge space, clean and surrounded by some green garden.Early morning moist,dew laden green grass, rising sun and cool fresh air made that space more refreshing. Few of my hospital staff, few enthusiastic patients started doing rounds regularly to our yoga garage at 6am. Starting from Aum to simple Asanas and to end with 15 mins of meditation it involved it all and was a wholesome experience. Strong mind is the base of strong body and heart. Mental health is more important than physical health because mental illness is the root cause of all our physical illness.So give good thoughts and good food to your soul and you will see the different You i used to tell them all. And this lady krushnamai was the esteemed member of our 6am club,87 and still running strong.She used to get up early in the morning, clean her small house do her morning rituals and puja.Then she walks daily half a mile to get bunch of newspaper and distribute it to the dozen of houses. After that she comes to yoga class do

Asanas actively,meditate with deep breath. As class comes to an end she opens her big thermas containing hot tea with special ginger elaichi taste and distributes to all. She sits for a while talking with me rather sharing her life experiences and touch our lives with her wisdom. She was our confession box to whom everyone can share everything and she had answers for all.She has amazing skills of convincing people by her talk.She was shoulder to cry and trusted place to lean over for emotional and mental support.She used to tell us many inspiring stories of her hard life,how she tackled her difficulties,how she fought her life's all odd. She was mother for many, guide and philosopher to all.She never got any formal education and never went to school but her knowledge came from the university of mother Nature.She learnt her lessons under the large open sky, her hard life was her ring master and with her strong will and determination she emerged as an all time university topper.

She was alone but not the lonely one. She had acquired many relationship based on her loving nature and care for all. Any one sick or ailing she visits them with hot home made food packed in her box.She gives them reiki therapy and some home remedies which she has learnt ages ago from her mother,grandmother and mother in law. Her warm touch and compassionate talks healed everyone more faster than any medicine. Born in a huge joint family, staying in a small house with dozens of siblings she was made to look after her young brothers and sisters and cousins when their parents went off to work in the fields.She was foster mother taking care of her siblings.Married off in a very young age she suffered number of abortions, home deliveries made her weak and fragile.Her husband lost his job from cotton mill and remained unemployed forever. Dived in addiction,drinking and abusing became his daily habit.She was subjected to daily domestic violence and physical abuse. With so many co morbidities her husband suffered many illnesses,got paralysed and was bedridden for a long time.But like an obident wife she kept taking care of her husband till his last breath.She worked as sweeper in our hospital and went to many houses for cleaning utensils and for other household works.But in her hard times also she was very positive, spoke well and was spik and span clean at her work.She never cried for attention nor gained sympathy telling her sob stories.But she was left totally broken when she lost her only son at a very young age.Her whole world toppled upside down.But if she looses herself she is not krushnamai...

After some days she shrugged off her grief and stood taller than before.Keeping her agonies buried deep in her heart she became Mai of everyone.She joined our hospital full time and spent her time with ailing patients giving them confidence and boosting their morale.At 11am she used to come with huge thermos filled with tea and distributed freely to all the attenders in the waiting hall.She used to sit and talk to them and shared their grief and pain. Sometimes she was seen consoling the irritable baby in the night sitting with baby's young mother,other time she was seen massaging the old lady patient's feet with oil, sometimes she was seen with school kid changing his forehead patti to bring down his fever,other time she could be seen talking with old grandpa and sharing his worries and making him feel better.In the afternoon she used to cook fresh simple food of hot rice, dal and vegetables and gave to all patients and their relatives.She never used to charge anyone but every one or other person gave her raw vegetables, dal, rice,oil and other ingredients to prepare her tasty meals everyday.She believed in "Vasudev kutumbakam" that means whole world is her family.She was an universal phenomenon and ubiquitous in our campus.Her food was so tasty that sometimes we used to keep our lunch boxes aside and gorge on her freshly prepared home food.

She made herself strong and started practising yoga at the

age of 60. She ate only twice and that too simple food of jowar roti and vegetables.She kept praying and helping others. At age of 87 she was standing strong with good health and super power memory. She inspired many to remain healthy and she taught us to care more for our mind and soul.She fasted twice a week and ate only fruits. It's neccesary for Soul Detox she used to say.Daily she walks few miles distributing Newspapers and milk.Keep yourself busy was her mantra.She was a lone warrior yet she strive hard to keep herself fit and healthy.

Mai why you work so hard at this age? You can rest for a while..We will look after the things, I used to say her. No my child , I'm fit because I'm working. I'm alone and I dont want to be burden on anyone. I try doing all healthy things because not that i want to live healthy but because I want to die healthy she said innocently. Die Healthy ?? What's that i raised my brows as it was a totally new concept for me. Look my child we all are going to die one day or other.No one can escape this universal truth. But if i get sick,ill and bedridden who will take care of me.Even if our keiths and kins are there to take care of us,its financial and mental burden on them.Morever we will torture our body and organs.So i strive hard to keep myself busy and occupied and eat healthy.

I pray to the God to pick me up instantly so that none of my people around has to feel burdened with my things.We can't write our fate, no one knows how we will die but atleast everyone should try their best for this.Everyone wants to live healthy but our goal should be to die healthy so everyone around us including we ourselves will be at peace.She was enlightening me. From where she gets soo much of wisdom i said to myself. I turned my head and saw her distributing a hot cup of tea to the patient attenders with a smiling face. She was no doubt everyones Mai... everyone's happy place.! Die Healthy... Seriously...it kept echoing in my ears and mind. This is what we all should strive for...i said to myself and walked positively for my work. Really a conversation with such amazing people will teach you things which 100 books cannot. My head bowed to this independent evergreen young girl in late 80's and my respect for her multiplied by thousand folds.

* * *

CHAPTER 14
HYDERABADI PATIENT NAWAJI

I love my profession and really i do. While treating various babies with variety of illnesses we come across variety of patient attenders and dealing with them we get lifetime experiences.Majority attenders and parents are nagging,irritating, anxious, argumentive, never satisfied with treatment nor explanation.Some are hyperactive,overtly emotional, always worrisome and always doubtful but nonetheless few people are grateful too.Sitting in my OPD and daily dealing with these kind of characteristic people with different attitude and nature I'm sure I will be pro at cracking PHD in psychology just in one go! Some patients are so irritating that we always want to avoid them or escape from them and some people are so Atarangi and funny that we will have our lungs out laughing and remembering consultation with them forever.

Arsalan....my opd sister called out the name opening the door. It was the call Bell for the next patient as inside patient goes out.Hearing to the name my face immediately frowned. I said sister order some hot cup of tea for me as i knew my 30 to

45 minutes were gone now as this patient of mine was very well known to be brain Eater to all, all the time.

Helloo Doctor madam kaise hai? Asma, Arsalan's mother, tall hefty lady creeped in through the small opening of my OPD door pushing the OPD sister outside. Clad in the full black full length burkha only thing to identify her was her heavy voice. Behind her came Arsalan busy eating some kurkure from half emptied packet.I don't know how many nth num of packet he might have binged on sitting outside my OPD. Followed by him came her cousin brother in early 20's who always accompanied them.This Trio was Foster family of our hospital as they make n number of trips to our hospital regularly with their infinite number of complaints and health issues which never existed in the child but they always felt it other way round like that in the Drishyam movie.!

Soo tell mi Asma,What's happening with Arsalan,how is he doing? There was nothing to be asked like this.Their bullets of questions used to keep firing randomly creating hyperbola to parabola and then used to be bola bola bola till i show them thombola. Patients like this will make you memorise your entire pediatrics in one go! Kuch pucho nakko madamji, haibaith haibath hori mereku ich isko dekh k...kuch khataich nahi she started.I was amazingly looking at the packets of kurkure, lays, Bourbon, cadburys which his uncle was giving him one after another and he was enjoying binging on it.21/2 yrs and 15 kgs, weight was good. Dont worry jitna khata hai khilao,weight toh accha hi hai i said. kya batao madam,khata khata khataich hai,phir wokariya kartaich rehta.Wak Wak bolta.kuch hazamich nahi hota isko.kuch hazme ki dawa likho.Hazam nahi hota toh baar baar toilet ich jaata yeh,aise khata,aise khata ki khateich toliet ko ich bhagta yeh.Aise khate hi bhagta ki pucho nakko.kuch motion rukne ki dawa dedo.Aur motion bhi dekho madamji kabhi patla hota, kabhi peela,kabhi harra, kabhi dono colour mix, smell toh aisi aati ki kuch puccho nakko saara mahuala puchta Arsalan toilet kara kya bolke.Toh hazme ki dawaich likho Zara she continued. Hazam nahi hota toh weight nahi badta na but his weight gain is good i said.Khane mei kirkirich madam.Din bhar bhagta rehta, kuch khana bole toh ghanta ghanta baiththa muah mei pakad kar she told his eating story.Par mere samne toh 2 packets chips, Bourbon, Cadbury abhi toh khaya 5-10 minutes mei hi i said surprisingly.Wohich pasand usko madam....kuch pucho mat...ghar ka bole toh kuch choothа bhi nahi.Daily pizza, burgers,Maggie ich hona isko.khata khata phir pet mei dard bolta....phir toilet ko gaya toh 1-1 ghanta toilet hotaich nahi isko.she continued her saga.Ab toilet hone ki dawa Dena ya toilet bandh hone ki likhna woh bolo i said bit annoyingly.Donoich likho ji ....jo lagta woh daalenge usko dawai she said. I now was feeling like banging my head. This is not evidence based medicine. This is convinence based medicine as per Patient's demand.

Parso bukharich aaya ji isko toh kaise kaise ki hora tha.Saas lene mei bahut taklif thi.Toh wahi pass Wale doctor ko ich dikhaye.She forwarded me prescription of multiple doctors ranging from Rmp, Unani, homeopathy, allopathy, childern specialist and what not.I just turned the various prescription pages only to find out another pediatrician writing only saline nasal drops for his so called serious saas lene mei taklif wali bimaari. Itte sabkon ko dikhaye? I asked shockingly. I was started feeling silly about myself by now. Whom i was thinking my very old patient whom I was seeing from birth thinking that they are my loyal patient and hence tolerating their ranting for hours together was found to be doctor shopping with every small and big clinician at the old city. Hou bahutich emergency hogayi thi madamji, idhar phone Kiya toh aap nahi hai bole. Leave pe gaye bole,toh haibath haibath hogayi.kisi ki bhi dawa laggich nahi isko. Har roj ek ek doctor ko mil k aaye.kya ji par aapki dawa chod k kuch jamtaich nahi isko, she told confidently.Soo full of gratitude my patients are to me i thought to myself.

Ok...toh ab kya hora isko, exact problem batao i said bit sternly.Bukharich nahi uttarra madam ji. Woh Numaish hoke aaye parso.Udhar woh colourwala barf ka gola khaya dekho tabse bukharich Chad Gaya isko.Aisa Aisa kaap Raha tha yeh pucho nakko....halak mei bhi dard hora tha. Kuch nahi khara tabse she added some more info. It reminded me that the most Famous yearly Exhibition of Hyderabad "' Numaish" has started. Kabse hai yeh problem i asked her.Parso se ich start hua, her innocent answer. Here parso in Hyderabad has very vast and deep meaning.Parso can be two weeks earlier or a day before or yesterday or may be two days later also. Here all the days except today is parso and this you will know only once you are hard core Hyderabadi. I started examining him keeping my palm on his stomach doing per abdomen examination to find out his pain.Idhar hai kya dard i asked this small Pokemon, poking packets and enjoying his treats which he got for coming to the hospital. Pet k thoda upar ji..halak mei dard hai isko.....she instantly pointed my ignorance in Urdu. Halak bole toh? i made question mark face.Gala ji..his uncle corrected me, thinking how dumb i was not knowing what halak means staying in Hyderabad. Ohh i said but neither he has fever,cold or cough.

His breathing is smooth and lungs are clear i told my points.Nahi maa bahutich tej bukhara tha isse, aisa khas ra tha ki pura halakhich bahar aata ki kya lagra tha.Toh emergency mei pass k doctor ko dikhaye toh dawa daale but abhi bhi kuch kamich nahi lagra.Aapki dawaich jamta isko she again started my praise chapter.Instantly his uncle removed 6-7 bottles consisting of 2 antibiotics, 2-3 varities of cough syrups, 2-3 varities of decongestants.Itta saara daal ri dekho iski ammi isse dawaaiya...phir bhi kuch bhi asarich nahi aara.I was shocked to see soo much stock of medicine being given for no actual problem. Kab se dere yeh dawai?i asked.Parso se ich ji their stock answer.Ohk yehi dawai continue Karo aur 3 days kam hojata.I was now fed up with their doctor shopping and over the counter medicine use.

Madamji woh last time aap calcium diye the woh continue karna kya she asked me showing her memory skill.Paira bahut dard marte ji iska, din bhar khelta khleta rehta ek zarra bolke nahi rukta, phir raat ko nahi sota, rota rehta full zor se, paira dukh re bolke....woh calcium daalu na phir....uss time daalke bandh kar diye the.Ok daalo no issue, but Kiku band karre? Now my accent was getting slowly old city style with Kiku..daldo and all the patent old city words creeping in my talk.Nahi madam ji, woh aap likhe the na calcium woh pineapple flavour tha, par inno pineapple nahi khata, mouj pasand inko.Toh woh baju gali Wale doctor banana flavour likhe toh pi liya yeh.Toh sardich hogayi isko,phir mouj khane se Sardi hori bolke woh bhi band kare.Par haddiyon mei se tarra tarra tarra awaz aari dekho iske,kuch calcium ki bhi dawa likh doh she added to his next misery.I was getting mad by this time.I wanted to yell and tell banana, pineapple are only flavours. Jaise gulab jamun mei gulab nahi hote vaise hi banana flavour syrup mei banana nahi hote.Par inn dedh dimagwalon ko kaun samazaye!

Madamji....isko bahut thakan hoti hai takat ki bhi dawa likh do jara,she again added to his list of unending complaints.Yeh kya last time yeh likh k diye na Bevon,wahi dedo i said frowningly.Woh kya hai ki madam ji woh dawai se washroom yellow yellow aara tha isko isliye woh band kar diye.Phir woh pass Wale doctor strawberry ki likhe takat ki dawa,par aapke Siva kuch jamta hi nahi isko dawai, jara kuch toh bhi likh do ji takat ki dawa she added.Now it was my time to get mad and start ranting at her.But our profession teach us to be patient with such limited edition specimen which check our patience to the core.

Madamji iske naak se khoon aata dekho baar baar.Aise aata

Aisa aata ki pura moosi tak ich chale jaata iska khoon.His uncle's neuronal sim suddenly got activated now (for those who don't know, Moosi is Hyderabad's famous river).Nose picking is the common reason for epistaxis in children i told them.Avoid nose picking and apply some pressure there for few minutes i guided them although I was boiling furiously from within by now.Vitamin C ki tablets likhri hun woh dena daily ek night ko i advised them.Vitamin C woh orange wali goli kya? mother asked curiously.Woh covid ke time sabko hi di the woh baju gali Wale doctor, par kya hai na madam ji isko orange colour pasand ich nahi hai dekho.Kuch green colour hai toh likh do ji Zara tablet she enlightened me.Now i was thinking we should have pediatric medicine shop like kirana shop outside our OPD's with tablets available in multiple colours and syrups available in various flavours.Jisko jo pasand woh lele!! Madam ji pressure daalo bolre naak pe..kisse daalna rumaal se kya? uncle's brilliant mind started working now.Hau kerchief se hi daal sakte i told in his language.Chota ya bada kerchief woh bhi boldo zara he asked me.Aare Miya... chota, bada, medium, white,grey, blue, plain, designwala jo pasand ho ya jo mile lelo ji.I answered him weiredly.We have to act weird like them at times with these wierd patient attenders.And may be that is the reason they get instantly connected with us.

Madamji woh parso aap tikon ka bole the na, woh dena hai ab they updated me.Now when this parso was i have to find out from their immunisation card.I opened their card only to know I have advised MMR vaccine at 9 months and from 9 months of age till 21/2 years their parso was not yet over and they haven't taken any vaccine from then.I was now getting angry, Yeh toh 9 months ka vaccine hai,ab tak kyun nahi liya? I asked furiously.Isko jab bhi vaccine dene ka time aata yeh bimarich hota.Ab last month ich laana tha but bukarich aagaya so nahi aaye they told easily.kitte dawa daale toh bhi utarich nahi tha bukhar.yeh daale the dekho isko,uncle took out one more bottle out of his pocket.One more antibiotic...ohh gosh...i was totally fed up by now.Kitne din se dere yeh? i asked with my last quota of patience.Ek mahine se dere phir bi kuch bhi kamich nahi hora isko,bukhar aara jaara aara jaara they explained their drug details.Ek mahine se i literally screamed.Ek mahine se antibiotics dere isko?kisne bola i was getting mad by now.Woh bukhar utarraich nahi tha toh mai ich di usko she uttered unshaken.I screamed now aisi kaunsi bimari hai jisko ek mahina antibiotics dena padta?kuch bimari nahi hai usko...acha khasa kha ra idhar samne baithk.Temperature normal hai, weight gain accha hain, physical growth development pura sahi hai uske age k liye.Kuch dawai mat do usse.koi jarurat nahi, khana khane se jyada dawaich kha ra woh i said angrily.Haanji madam sahi pakade, kuch khataich nahi woh.Bhook hi nahi hori usko.Bhook ki koi dawa likho she added one more to her farmaish."Sab band kardo dawai uski.Pura normal hai woh...koi dawai ki jarurat nahi"i shouted at them.Looking at my angry gesture uncle said ok madam tika likhdo leke aate abhi.Now..??? I almost screamed.It's 6 past already my OPD time is over.Next time lelo 2-3 days k baad aake i told them reluctantly.

Nakko ji madam aisa nakko karo, abhich leke aata mai, pehleich Zara der Hui na tika dene he asked in pleading tone.Zara der??? Bhaiye it's more than 1 n half year ka der, i thought to myself.Hyderabadi nawab na yeh sab.Inke time se aate doctor se milne,inke convience se treatment hona, ab laate vaccine ,doctor should wait extra time post their OPD hours for their vaccination. Nawab log gaye Hyderabad se par inki Nawabi nahi gayi abtak i mumbled to myself. I waited impatiently for another 20 minutes for him to get his vaccine.20 minutes later my OPD sister peeped inside and said madam unko kuch doubt hai Kate,baat karte Kate she informed me in her broken Urdu mixed Hindi.Bhej do I told frowning.

Now uncle entered holding vaccine prescription, followed by Arsalan eating now banana(called mouj in Hyderabad)followed by his mother.Woh kya hai na madam ji utta amount Zara Kam hai iss time, woh aap bole jaisa parosoich laake lagwata mai vaccine.Zara kuch bhi nakko samzo iss time they informed me their plight.Ok i said controlling my anger for wasting my soo long and precious time. I took my bag and fleeted hurriedly out of my OPD leaving a big sigh of relief as i knew their parso will be after many months now.

Tomorrow they will be at some other clinic telling them kaisa kaisa ki toh hora isko...aapki dawa chod k kuch lagtaich nahi. I kicked my bike with full force to vent out all my frustration of 45 minutes of long conversation which was mentally tiring and exhausting for me.Fresh air outside made me feel like some release phenomenon making myself very light.And i started laughing reminding all the Scenario with hare ,Peele n orange tablets.Pineapple,banana strawberry syrups.I laughed out loud saying halak k upar ka kamra than dhan than bolke dard karra mera, sarr futt ra mera, garma garam chai daal lena ab halak mei and i started laughing to myself. Baigana jaise kya baata karri hun mai.Ab toh mai bhi ban gayi pakka hyderabadi.!! To tolerate such patients one requires heights of patience and to talk to them with great elan at their next visit needs some miraculous power. And these kinds of miracles keeps happening to me all the time in my medical practice giving me booster energy to welcome them again with a hello Arsalan kaise ho and then followed by kya batau madamji kaise kaise ki hora.....and then...the cycle continues...!!!

* * *

CHAPTER 15
BRAVE HEARTS

It was early 2020.We were just back from our Singapore-Thailand trip and then was this Havock.Covid had hit India and was on the rise marking the beginning of pandemic.New year had started on a bang but on a very scary note,Novel virus...rapid spread... thousands of lives on stake.One state to another,one country to another and within no time entire world was affected. Borders were closed,transport and interstate travel was shut down and the entire world came to a complete halt.Lockdown was announced and the World was seized.People were confined to their small houses,neighbours became alien,maid's were waved off.Years together maid dependant women suddenly became self sufficient.Dinners,Outings and get togethers became just once upon a time things and human relationships were on the verge of extinction.Whole universe was on topsy turvy.

Slightest cold, cough and fever brought spine chilling thoughts.Entire families were getting affected.Long queues in the OPD,maddening crowds...Every one wanted admission to the hospital.Even single denial for admission was getting outrageous. Suddenly doctors were the most sought after.Till now the one who were abused, criticised as money minting and gold diggers suddenly were given the Godly status.Oxygen was the costliest air,lack of beds,lack of oxygen, more and more patients and lack of infrastructure. The health care system totally collapsed and the entire medical fraternity was completely exhausted attending to the endless patients. People abandoned their own Keith's but Doctors were considered as emotional Robots to serve people relentlessly under the name of noble profession and humanity.Doctors were leading the orphan's life without meeting their kids,spouses,parents for weeks together.

They have left their homes and were staying aloof in the hospital shelters.The fear of contracting this deadly virus and spreading it to their loved ones made chills running down their spines.We all were on a Mission...draped in full gowns, masks,caps and gloves 24/7, feeling drenched with sweat,suffocated with lack of oxygen, breathing through the thick masks and heavy respirators having hypoxic feeling but yet maintaining aseptic decorum.We were living into a different time zone...no contact with outer world,not seeing rising or setting sun.How many died and how many were saved, how many still alive holding their breaths...Newspaper flashed it daily but we remained unaware in these closed ICU's treating patients and trying to get them back to life.

Some one's Father was in the icu....someone's mother was in the ward. children were waiting in their homes with eager eyes to see their parents. Old grandparents were staying worried in their villages trying to get information about their daughters,sons and grand kids.It was no doubt a wierd world and a heart rendering situation.Entire universe was divided into barriers,different zones, different borders, different sections,icu's,wards and home isolation. Who will be there tomorrow and who won't was the question.

. . .

We were packed in our thick disposable gowns with only a small window kept open at our eyes to see the outer world.Double masks and gloves were our guards."Madam some lady is at our hospital door step,looking full term in labour pains,she is breathless"our duty doctor in ER called me on the icu intercom.Labour room was jamm packed,many women with ongoing labour pains were in waiting, routine Lscs were conducted in regular OT.Now where to accommodate her? I started thinking.

Hospital PRE went to enquire about her.She was breathing heavily,her temperature was high,she was rolling in pain.It was no doubt an emergency...two lives were at stake.Her symptoms suggested covid. We cannot take her in the routine operation theatre,her Rt PCR will take time our doctor on duty was reminding me of the current situation.I told to shift her in casualty first,she needs to be examined. She is in active labour...where can we send her in this situation? More than a doctor,a woman in me was speaking.We couldn't see any of her attenders around.We pulled her on the trolley and shifted her to ER. Her previous cesarean scar was very thin,fragile and about to give away.We need to operate her urgently our gynaecologist informed us. Suddenly there was grin,unbooked case mam, don't know her other virological status(Hiv, HbsAg), RT PCR won't come so early, even her attenders are not seen around... our doctors in ER started showing reluctance to take this case which has come at the very last moment.Their worries were really relevant and true.But i was very sure if not we now then she would not survive.

I convinced our gynaecologist,she being senior most and most respectable doctor in the town understood the real situation.Shift her to septic OT she instructed ER staff.And then followed the 30 minutes thrill drill where everyone started working on the war foot.Rapid test was done in ER, it was positive so we need to be extra careful. Everyone was ready in their sterile disposable scrubs, double masks, gloves.she was made ready with cannula in situ, IV Fluids and shot of antibiotic. Blood tests were sent on the emergency basis,CT chest was done which showed Corad 5, means definitely covid.Now as we all have taken this challenge we have to keep going... there was no chance to turn around.

We have to operate her under GA our experienced gynaecologist instructed the anaesthesist seeing her general condition. She was quickly intubated and sedated.Lungs were taken care of...the critical care team took control of BP and vitals and skillful obstetric team was quick to deliver.Within 8 minutes baby was on the rescucitation bay in front of me lying listless and blue.She wasn't breathing.My Neonatal rescucitation skills came into play,i pumped the artificial breaths into her lungs... bit of colour and heart rate improved but breathing was not smooth.Baby developed severe distress and i had to intubate her on table.We shifted the baby to isolation zone and started on ventilator,her lungs showed pneumonic patch and blood test showed severe infection.We treated her with the best possible treatment covering good antibiotics,cardiorespiratory support and ionotropes.Fresh frozen plasma and platelets were infused in view of cogaulopathy.After battling for over 10 days for life baby started slowly improving.Her vitals stabilized and she was weaned off to the room air gradually from ventilator and CPAP.Slowly she started accepting spoon feeds.

On the other side gynaecologist were trying hard to save the mother.She was given papinavir and remdisivir, the drugs used in covid,she was ventilated for 4 days and slowly weaned off.Now she was better and was shifted to the room.We transferred the baby to the mother and Ahhh what an emotional moment it was! Mother hugged the baby and weeped in joy.This scene was so joyous in the four closed walls. Although there were barriers and they were isolated from the rest of the world they seemed to be so happy being together after so many days.Mother told that her entire family suffered from covid and were hospitalised to the government hospital and she wasn't aware how they were. All her relatives abandoned them. She was set into labour in the night and no one came for her rescue. She alone walked in the night from her Village to reach our hospital and she collapsed at our door step.She knew her pregnancy would be critical and she has to travel to higher centre if she wants to survive herself and her baby.She thanked all of us for the great help, the tears of joys and happiness kept rolling on her cheeks continuously.

We informed her family members at Government hospital.Her husband was recovering in the ward, her in laws were on the verge of getting discharged.As they were getting stable their few relatives came to see them. Grandparents along with two relatives reached our hospital.Holding the baby in their hand the old couple weeped a lot.You are not like God but you are the God for us....their voice trembled as they came forward to touch my feet.No no just thanks the Almighty.He is the creator and He is the protector i said."we were very scared madam as many of our village people succumbed to this illness and even their family members couldn't attend their last rites.We thought meeting these people if we contract this disease we and our family would be in trouble " their relatives tried explaining and justifying their act.When their own family members and relatives disowned them we doctors were giving our best to save them.The thrill of taking challenges and giving one's best in tough and life threatening condition is what makes Medical field above all.

Next day both, the mother and the baby were ready for discharge.All came to meet me in my cabin.The old elderly Village clad in-laws and the baby with her mother were standing in front of me.What about fees madam? they asked me worriedly.Looking at them i could easily make out they were not in position to pay any of our bills.I have told our hospital to create some free slots for extremely needy patients to tackle emergency situations like these till covid gets over on humanitarian grounds and we have treated this patient under such one slot.Sometimes earning blessings is more important than earning money and this pandemic has taught everyone to be the humans first.

Yeah surely you have to pay our bill i said seriously.They looked helpless.How much madam? her father in law asked in tearful voice." One cup of tea" when i come to visit you i said smilingly.They were stunned and amazed by my answer."Ohh sure sure madam...why only tea you come over lunch.You have done so much for us,we are lifetime indebted to you" and all the three started crying.No worries God sent her here and we just helped her doing our duties i said calmly. "God bless you Mam" they said heartfully.My all bills and dues were instantly cleared with their heartfelt blessings.They walked out of my room beaming with their little bundle of joy.All our staff clapped for them in the corridor. I saluted all my colleuges, doctors, nursing staff who sacrificed their lives to treat all these critical patients in the pandemic.They all are true Bravehearts...the frontline warriors like our Indian army on the border saving our countrymen. "Party tonight for everyone from my side"i announced and all the bravehearts started smiling and clapping with more energy.The ward echoed with more joys now!!!!

* * *

CHAPTER 16
LAST SUPPER

Atlast OPD over.I jumped with joy and hurriedly ran towards the car parking of our government hospital at Miraj,opened my car door,sat on the driver seat,fastened my seat belt getting ready for a joy ride! The loud music was on as soon as I started my car, long list of do's on the weekend was ready.Finally a free weekend for which I was waiting eagerly for so long.One and a half day of well deserved break after such a long working full month.I was thinking about my holiday list.Will just go home, enjoy Pet full (stomach full) and heartful of garmagaram meal and sleep as if there is no tomorrow.Get up for a hot cup of tea with snacks and binge watch on these melodramatic TV serials.Sometimes these saas bahu operas are so entertaining.Sunday is funday loaded with outings, shopping, eating in my favourite food joints, catching up with some friends and watching some good movie in the theatres.Hustly bustly weekend and I was ready,just to pull the trigger.I was lost in my dreamy thoughts when suddenly loud voice rukkooo... banged on my ears and my leg pressed the brakes hard.

A small boy of 3 years bent behind my rear wheel,took out

his brown puppy,raised his hands and showed me shaking the puppy.

“Family" he again roared angrily as he was annoyed as i did not watch out for his puppy while taking the reverse for my car.I peeped out of my window and said "Sorry Dost dekha nahi."He replied "dyan se, next time. I got out of my car, caressed his little soft furry brown ball and said pakka.Now there was a sigh of relief on that little boy's face and he went dancing keeping his little puppy on his head. Really family is not about blood always i said to myself.Next two days i was busy enjoying my holidays and totally forgot about this incidence.

Monday morning i was hurrying towards our pediatric ICU for rounds when I saw this same fair little boy playing with his dog in our car parking and a few other boys and girls lying down nearby under the shade of tree busy in their own little world.Why all these people are here i entered ICU wondering.They all look typical Rajasthani Marwaris from their dressing and attires i guessed.

Mam this boy was admitted on Saturday evening.He is irritable,agitated with increased tone in all the four limbs.Our PG's on rounds updated me.And he is Rajasthani i mumbled.My PG's were shocked and shook their heads in a big yes! Now i got the link.This boy belonged to the family who were waiting outside in our hospital verandah.I examined him thoroughly.He was robust young boy 13 yrs old, tall,fair but deeply sedated.His whole body was getting rigid and tight slowly and his breathing was abnormal.Many wires and cables were hanging around his body. He was breathing through NRM mask. IV fluids lines, ECG cables, oxygen pipes, pulse oximeter were showing his criticality.I ordered the treatment and turn around to speak to the family.My diagnosis was almost done!

So kitne saal se ho yaha,kya kaam karte ho idhar?I enquired his basic details.His older sibling hardly 17 years old came forward. "7 saal se hai, yeh Bhai Mera Jo aapka patient hai,bas 6 saal ka tha tab" he told me silently looking lost. Bahar jo sab hai aap hi ke log hai kya? My curiosity was unending."Haanji madam,sab bhai behen hai mere.Total 7 log hai hum, mai bada 17 saal ka hun, yeh aapka patient 3 number and sab se chota wala 3 saal ka hai.Maa hai humare saath, pita gujar gaye. Thekedaar leke aaya hume kaam pe, seth ka mithai bhandar hai.Hum mithai banate hai udhar, seth two time ka khana deta hai and ek room hai sone ko. Baki kaam k paise thekedaar rakh leta hai" he said with a grin.I felt so sorry to know the hands which were making sweets and filling sweetness in others life,their own life was so bitter.Life is really so unfair to some!

School gaye kabhi?i asked him.Nahi madam, he chukled. Uss sab k liye time kaha? My diagnosis was almost confirmed with this brief conversation now.kabhi koi tika lagwaya hai? I bounced him with my last question.Nahi, Rajasthan ke bahut chote gaav se hai hum log, koi haspatal nahi udhar, peene ko pani nahi milta,dawai milna bahut durr ki baat hai madam he said looking into the hollow.Bhai kaisa hai mera madam? he asked with painful voice.

The tension and the worry masked his face. Taking his socioeconomic history i have concluded my diagnosis. He is very sick,breathing fast, irritable, body getting rigid, today he is able to eat and drink a bit but i don't know about tomorrow how he will be I explained him sadly.He almost choked.Kya bimari hai yeh? he asked with a trembling voice.Tetanus...ek type ka infection hai.Home delivery, unclean instruments, unhygienic conditions and moreover not vaccinating kids is the main reason why the children get this i told him in the easiest possible language which he can understand. But i feel more sorry because i know this disease is preventable with just a small prick of injection called vaccine i updated him.

Will he be saved? his eyes were tearful. I engulfed my sadness, "we will try our best but chances look bleak. May be he will require to put on ventilator" i said empatheticly which my profession has taught me over these many years. He started crying wanting to see his ailing brother.He went into the ICU, sat next to him holding his hand.His younger brother opened his eyes,trying to fake a smile. Bhai kya laaye mere liye? he asked innocently,unaware of his illness.He turned his face towards the side and started sobbing.After sometime he walked to me, Madam ek puchna tha he asked politely.Kya hai bolo? i looked puzzled.Ek aakhari baar saath mei khana kha sakte hai kya hum sab log? his voice broke me down.My tears started rolling listening to his question.I nodded my head in a yes.He gathered his family near to the ICU window. Elder sibling went out,he served them food, waah halwa those all other younger siblings screamed unaware of their brother's condition in the ICU.This halwa was probably the last dinner they were going to eat together.He got some halwa in the plate,fed his ailing sick brother with lots of love and care but he hardly could swallow it.This was the real painting of real family eating together their last meal.More surreal than the Da Vinci's world famous painting on the Last Supper! It touched my heart deeply and i had traumatic impact of this on my mind.I couldn't sleep the entire night.

Next day with a heavy heart I entered the ICU only to find his bed empty. There is nothing to be told about the empty beds in the government hospital ICU's.They speak volumes about themselves.We ventilated him at midnight but couldn't save him despite all our efforts, Dr Wasnik Night incharge doctor of our ICU updated me. Till then the same 3 years old boy with his dog on his head came with his eldest brother to me unaware of what has happened to his other brother last night. "Family" he screamed looking at me reminding me the car wheel incidence of his puppy under my car. He shook his dog and showed him to me.I kept my hand patting his furry back unable to talk to them."Madamji....jaa rahe hai hum ab but 10 days k baad inn sabko leke aata hun.Tika lagwado inn sabko" and he started weeping badly. I too couldn't hold my tears back. Atlast I'm human too!!

I turned my head towards the window and could see the whole family walking out of the hospital gate.The big Banyan tree under shades of which the entire family stayed for 4-5 days looked orphan now!!

Simple vaccine awareness could have saved this life i uttered to myself. In this advanced Era of Vaccination loosing a child for preventable disease like Tetanus was failure of the entire system i felt.Despite extensive vaccine drives and mop ups still getting to see Tetanus in 21st century was soo disheartening.Vaccine awareness is very important to prevent this avoidable diseases. But still some places in India are unreached and far from getting acquainted with basic things like education and basic medical facilities.For them earning daily bread and butter and feeding their big families is the biggest battle to win! But just a small jab would have saved this young life i thought to myself.Their Last supper got etched in my mind forever like the Da Vinci's one..!!!

* * *

CHAPTER 17

PURSUIT OF HAPPINESS

What a movie! I exclaimed as I pressed the sleep button on my P. C after seeing the most heart touching end of the Pursuit of happiness past midnite.And I could not erase Will Smith's, Chris Gardener in the movie.What a role played man...so simple yet so strong and so effective.I always believe "All work and no play makes Jack a dull boy"! And hence I try to make some time for myself daily where I go for movies and enjoy the larger than life 70mm drama or visit a new restaurant or cafe in the city with thrilling ambience and tickle my tastebuds orelse read a book with my mouth wide open with protagonist giving a surprising twist in the story or wheeling around the woods exploring the

new places or sometimes just spread myself on a sofa leisurely watching the most entertaining saas bahu daily soap operas on our very own Tv. I enjoy anything and everything till it relaxes my body and mind and refreshes my soul.And with this movie I ticked my one more bucket list wish.This movie may not have garnered the Oscar but no doubt have won millions of hearts.Feeling of joy and sadness admixed rolled over my cheeks when I snoozed in my warm blanket while the thought of pursuit of happiness kept lingering on me all over the night till the very next morning.

Bang..Bang...Bang the hatrick sound of our three Nicu doors from the main door to the level three Nicu room marked the arrival of a new baby in the Nicu. Cutting short our morning rounds and case discussion with our PG's we rushed towards our registrar who was getting a baby hurriedly with the sweating forehead.Tensly he said, baby did not cry at birth and required stimulation and oxygen so got here and in no time we could understand how hard time he would have had with the attenders to be in such a sultry state. He whispered slowly as he left the place briskly "Get ready for a new war as the attenders are naggingly aggressive." And then we could hear the loud thunderous voice of the baby's father and 3 other men in the village attire fighting with the security guard and trying to intrude in the Nicu.

I want my baby at any cost, do anything but save my baby he was shouting at high pitch.Orelse I won't spare anyone.He was as wild as wild cat. I took him inside and showed his baby who had irregular and jerky respiration with bad sensorium. I knew it was more of the brain involvement rather than the lungs.I told him to wait in the counselling room till we settle his baby and he looked bit convinced. I ventilated the baby, started necessary treatment.Tests were sent & brain scan was planned.Blood gas showed metabolic acidosis. I gave the required instructions to the nursing staff and reached the counselling room making up my mind as how to face this man.

By the time I reached the counselling room his wildness has mellowed down and this angry yelling man was now a soft hearted father. Looking at me he started weeping loudly."Save my baby mam, I have lost my earlier kid also on day 3 of life.I had travelled 350 kms from my village to the city but couldn't save my baby. Please save this baby at least"he said sobbing.

Emotional turmoil of the parents seeing their baby suffering at birth frequently turns them more violent and hostile.This is the time where we need to be really patient and understand their emotional needs.

I took the history and noticed that there was consanguinity(Marriage within the cousins), first child also did not cry, had fits, was ventilated and died at 3 days of life. So detailed evaluation was not possible that time.However Lactate report was elevated. We knew we were dealing with the genetic issue, more precisely with inborn error of metabolism in which some problems occurs if parents marriage is in close relation. As expected the routine blood investigations were normal but lactate was high.TMS and GCMS showed mixed acidemia where acid in the body increases many folds.We started the baby on the Metabolic Cocktail.Sodium bicarbonate infusion was continued uninterrupted but the acid levels remained very high.Genetic counselling was done to the father and genetic test was sent which also revealed genetic mutation leading to the acid disorder in the baby and it was supposed to pass on to the next generation as well.

To break this news to the already annoyed father was like a thunder bolt hitting hard.We explained him in detail how some diseases are related to the genes in our body and are transmitted to our kids as well. Most of these diseases are life threatening without any definitive cure. Father was totally disheartened but he seem to be getting on the terms slowly. Being a villager with a very miniscule income he tried his best to survive his kid. But sometimes destiny has other plans and fate plays the villian.

Days were passing but there were no signs of improvement.Baby was fighting for his every single breath but acid levels continued to remain high.And after a certain point, treatment modalities got exhausted and we came to the brutal reality of life.After consulting few more doctors in his area and after discussing with his friends,relatives and his family he came to me with painful heart and said "I did what so ever possible for my kid madam but God loves him more so he hasn't given any other option to keep this baby with me.I have realized this and have decided to take my baby home so that he can spend some moments with his mother for the last time.We respected his words and his decision and discharged the baby with a heavy heart.This was the same angry violent father on day one of admission who was now heart broken and cold. Some decisions are hard for the parents to make but more harder for any doctor to execute.

" Thanks madam for everything you did, you took very good care of my son.You explained the things clearly and transparently and helped me to understand the fact.I will never forget your help" he said emotionally while leaving.Some patients turns you sympathetic from being empathetic.At the end we doctors are humans as well !

And after a month I could see the same village cladden man waiting at my opd door. Please come in I said gently.He gave me a small invitation printed on thin blue paper."My son's Naamkaran madam..I want you to come and bless my child, please dont say No. I will be the happiest person if you come to attend our small function" he said softly.

Your son?when?how?? I was confused and lost.Looking at my question mark face he said, madam my own son passed away after a day we took him home. I was completely shattered as I knew we won't be having babies again. But then one of my relatives delivered this baby and they already had kids so we adopted this child.This baby is our new sunshine and he has brought lots of happiness in our lives.Now we are no more in the empty nest, this boy has filled all our world with joy.His face was bright and there were twinkle in his eyes.

. . .

And this is the meaning of pursuit of happiness I felt. This common man showed me, Happiness is largely a choice and not an entitlement. I was amazed to see how these simple people build their own life and discover their own path of fulfillment and wellbeing.This simple man taught me complex life lesson in a simpler way.He taught us how to embrace life with sorrows and joys.To accept the things as they are and not to crib or sulk in the past but to rise again like a Phoenix and chase the happiness.As we all know the happiness is a state of mind and we need to belive in the process.Finally it's truly said "Happiness is not a destination to arrive but a journey to travel!"And this man by his simple gesture has found his own way to pursue his happiness.Really sometimes these simple people make ordinary things to look extraordinary.And yes what most is needed for this extraordinary thing is just that small extra acceptance!!

* * *

CHAPTER 18

TWILIGHT SAGA: A SILENT NIGHT

Although being a doctor i always believe I'm gypsy at my heart. A gypsy of Merry land who always find time to go wherever i feel most alive.You can often find me smelling the sea, feeling the sky, chasing the waterfalls and getting into the woods close to nature where my soul rests and spirit fly!My profession takes me to various places and shows me Myriad of human emotions creating memories of Gold! And this one memory is dark, scary yet the one which made me stronger and richer in my experiences of what i love to do " Saving Lives"..!

It was our internship period where we have just come out of our bookish world and were trying our hands practically on the different diseases trying to cure them.As a part of rotation we were posted in the remote konkan area called kini where our college was running it's PHC (primary Health Center).Chasing our dreams and clearing the toughest course of MBBS, we arrived with handful of clothes and some necessary items in our back pack to this world of new adventures and started our show.

Small village with rough roads, white dust, dense forest like areas around, no proper transport facility with mere only one bus getting into the village daily.Sunrise lightening up the village and the sunset making it dark was the only time machine here.Smoky chullas clouding the sky preparing for the night dinner and at 9 pm the village used to be dead asleep.No much Mobile network, no hotels or no other entertainment places.Just get up,go to health centre,treat the patients with whatever small scale medicines available,wait for the results and moreover pray for the patient's wellbeing was all what we were doing here.Our hearts were full of hollow feelings and the mind full of insecurities but it was the place where i realised the power of prayers.When you have very little but could do the wonders.So the roller coaster ride was going on in this Kini PHC with varieties of people coming with different problems and we the amateur doctors trying different permutations and combination of our theoretical and practical knowledge to save them.

First day was as new as a fresh dew. I along with my Doctor twin sister and one of my other Batchmate were waiting eagerly to treat our very first patient.And here came a young man with fishing hook deeply rooted in his nail bed stuck hard, bleeding heavily and the person was wincing badly with pain.We applied local anaesthesia and tried all our surgical skills learnt in the surgery wards to remove that hook but our young energy was falling short.Then as it is said United we stand..we all three doctors took the long forceps,applied it to the hook and with all our mighty strength we pulled the hook out cheering Jai Bajrang Bali ki...and with loud cheer came out the huge hook stucked in his finger bed.That moment was as big as India winning the world cup final,that too against Pakistan.Our joys knew no bounds.We dressed his wounded finger artistically with all aseptic precautions, gave him a course of antibiotics and painkiller.And thus from here our journey of being Medical practitioner started in a real sense.

Days were passing by adding new patients, new diagnosis, new treatments and moreover new experiences to our kitty.It was here for the first time i learnt to give intramuscular injection, it was here i conducted the normal delivery and holding the just born baby for the very first time felt magical.I cannot forget umpteen number of attempts of doing, undoing n redoing practice of suturing before actual episiotomy suturing and then assessing our suturing skills indirectly by the style of patient's walk.Weekly twice we used to walk 10 kms in a deserted area listening to rustic music of fallen leaves to reach a small human habitat to either vaccinate newborns or to distribute iron and folic acid supplements to the pregnant ladies under various Bharath Sarkar Schemes.So this place was a real gurukul for us where we learnt zillions of new things daily.And yes we weren't just surviving here but living quiet a thrilling life.

In the evenings after hospital times, our PHC courtyard used to get converted into a badminton court and we all used to enjoy few hearty games.After tiring work the piping hot ginger tea and delicious pohe from Anju's hotel on the way back home used to be literally feast for us.Retiring on the cotton bed after long hectic hours of work used to be so peaceful and that small cottage rented for us by our hospital was like a Queen's Paradise!

But amidst all, One night was the most scariest and adventurous which is etched in my mind and memory forever. It was a deep,dark rainy night.Rain was pouring heavily since evening making the visibility of even few steps very difficult.Kokan is known for the heavy rains and once started it rains for days together without any break.We had our dinner early and were cuddling in our beds in the warm blankets,scared inside out but trying to fall asleep.No electricity and buzzing sounds of night insects was making the surrounding more lonely.

At midnight 2 some thumping sounds on our door got us out of our sleep.Some patient attenders were on the door calling us for the help.None of us had courage to get up and open the door.We looked at Balawwa,our caretaker who was the local woman who stayed with us and took care of our things.She got up, increased the light of the latern hanged up in one corner of the room and asked aloud what has happened? The people outside told that they have brought a patient with snake bite to PHC and he was sick and critical and needed our help.In such horrendous rains all the routes to city were blocked and they couldn't think of anything but about us.

Chill went down our spine listening to their story and we didn't know how to treat a snake bite except for reading it for our exams in our textbook.We were reluctant to open the doors but the Doctor inside us didn't calm down.Our emotional quotient got energezised.We wore our raincoats, took big torches in our hands, took umbrellas and walked out of the house.The pitch dark region, horrible rains breaking the serenity of surrounding, occasional dog howling in the freezing cold...and we doctors walking between the two troupes of the people going ahead and few behind us with torches in their hands and torch light showing us our way to the hospital.

Reaching the hospital we saw a person lying in a very critical stage on the patient bed. He had ptosis, altered sensorium and was going into shock with pale body and feeble pulse.Our young minds started at work.Urgently we secured an iv line, started him on oxygen, started him on iv fluids and medicines to maintain BP. Only now life saving drug was ASV (anti snake venom) which we have read in the books and knew the side effects of this drug were more horrifying than its effect.And chances of death of the patient with fear of snakebite was more than the drug itself.

We gathered courage and spoke to the attenders, told them that the patient was very sick and we cannot guarantee his life but can try our best."You are the only hope for us now madam try whatever you can"said the crowd unanimously. Their belief in us doubled our courage and boosted our morale.

One by one we broke the ASV ampoules,added it in iv fluid, started the drip and kept monitoring the patient entire night.The beeps of pulseoximetry moniters were breaking the entire silence.We were treating, monitoring and praying for the patient's survival.The crowd of 15-20 people accompanying him were praying in their respective religious manner.There was pindrop silence around but this silence spoke volumes.Every single minute passing was like a huge era and was racing our heart beats in heaps of anxiety.That was the night where i might have prayed to all 33 crores gods in total despair telling him to save that man and moreover to save our lives too.Our hopes of becoming world famous doctors would have shattered down to dust if this person would not have survived.Whole night we were wide awake with only thought that person should get revived back to the life.

Night waned and rain stopped.The golden showers started spreading on the blue sky,cool breeze eased the tension in the room and we could see his vitals on the monitor getting stabilised slowly.The ASV has done it's job.Heart rate normalised, blood pressure picked up and slowly that person opened his eyes.Whole crowd was thrilled with joy and the happiness on their faces just overflowed! We were too over joyous to say anything but our tears expressed our emotions.The whole hard work we have put in for the entire 5 years of learning medicine has paid off.The entire tanda came to us and greeted with gratitude.Today we got to know why Doctors are called next to God."We haven't seen gods in real but saw it today in you all" they said emotinally. That was our life's biggest achievement more valuable than any prize we have ever got.That was the day we realised that being a doctor is not just a profession but it's a special gift of imparting life.That aesthetic happiness and satisfaction we get in saving a life cannot be measured but only can be treasured.And from thereon our adventurous medical life began. So this is the story of the silent night which we literally lived and expirenced. Nevertheless to say the hot piping tea we had on that dawny morning was the best tea i have ever had in my life. That's why i said some Memories are just Pure Gold ! They cannot be erased but only can be etched forever.....Just like this one.!!!

* * *

CHAPTER 19
THE LOST TRIBALS

It was the time when i was working in the Primary health centre(PHC)amidst the dense green forest. It was a satellite centre of our main tertiary care hospital in the city which was a tribal land. We used to go by public transport till the small pathway which led into deep, rustic dense green forest.Walking the narrow pathway we used to reach the river bank and used to get onto the small boat which took us to the opposite river bank and walking for about half a mile was the small habitat of these locals.They used to speak different language and used to follow different and strange rituals.Their eye catchy dresses were made up of varities of leaves and colourful pieces of clothes, ladies used to wear thick off white bangles till elbows and mirror clad ghagra choli which was their traditional attire. Men used to put colourful feathered narrow ribbon like bands on their heads.They looked aliens to us and we looked aliens to them.

Earlier when we used to visit them along with the forest department police, there used to be lots of resistance and non-coperation.We used to travel in hot sun and heavy rains to reach their locality and wait whole day for them to come and visit us in our small clinic. But in our initial days to our dismay not a single person turned around. We could see them suffering and ailing.Many running high grade fever, children were often sick with variety of infections and usually succumbed to diarrhoea and Pneumonias.Many pregnant ladies died of deprived medical care, severe anemia and loss of blood.Dengue, malaria, rickettsial infections were very much common. But everytime they used to attribute it to some angry God and used to do various Puja and rituals sometimes getting better and sometimes losing their lives.They needed lots of education to make them understand that the infections are making them sick and moreover to make them believe that treatment does exist for it.

We got clubbed with the forest officers, local heads and started arranging meetings with those people. I understood if i need to make them believe me I have to learn their language first. I searched the entire Google and researched about this tribe, their customs, their language. Local heads helped me in this and slowly and steadily i learnt their language and now i could understand their feelings and needs in a better way and they too understood I'm their friend in their needs.As the faith built up they started coming slowly for their health aliments to our small clinic.We used to treat simple common aliments at their locality and used to shift sick cases to our tertiary hospital with our field workers.When they saw their own people getting alright they found it miraculous and now every one from the tribe were our regular visitors.For their every problem we had the solution and thus we turned into best friends from foe within few months.

They started calling us for their tribal functions.Most celebrated ones were like their God's fair (Jatra).They used to gather together and place their Goddess on the platform and used to dance in circles after performing Puja.They had their local instruments like drums,wind pipes and they used to sing and dance their heart out in these functions.I was fortunate enough to witness their some strange yet very different marriages and taste some of their local sweets and delicacies. Staying along with them and knowing about their traditions and customs i got to know they had high rates of inherited or genetic diseases as almost all of their marriages were within their tribe itself.

Among such illnesses one illness was bit different yet life threatening.We had this child of about 10 months who often presented with vomitings and loose motions.Earlier we thought of infections and treated him with the antibiotics but as the child was not improving we got him to the city to our tertiary care hospital.Blood tests revealed low potassium and ABG showed metabolic alkalosis.And now we were sure that we weren't dealing with some infections or any common aliments but it was a life threatening genetic disorder called as Gittelman's syndrome which required life long pottasium supplement. We counselled them regarding the problem and need of iv potassium and explained them regarding baby's long term prognosis.They started visiting us every fortnight for potassium supplements.We used to admit him, give iv pottasium,moniter the child and then discharge. Months after months child came and we started treating them for free looking at their financial condition. By now they too have understood that this is just a supportive and palliative treatment and child will not survive for long.

Like every fortnight this time also child came to us for iv pottasium.We checked him, inserted iv cannula and started the infusion.Child was looking sick from the past few visits.This time baby looked dehydrated with laboured breathing.We started him on the oxygen and potassium drip.Looking at his sinking condition we have often counselled them regarding the poor outcome and poor prognosis of this disease. I did my icu and ward rounds and came to Doctors room. It was 11 pm past and Dinner was already waiting for me in the Doctors room.My juniors were busy in the wards and ICU doing their rounds and monitoring the patients.I was about to start with my meal when a crowd of people started running haywire,there were screams,few people crashed into the doctors room and started rukus.Our child is dead...your junior did not do anything...they were shouting at the top of their voices.I could hear the sounds of smashing things from the ICU. I ran barefooted to see what was happening.A large crowd was busy destroying things in and outside the icu, they were pushing our junior doctor aside. I squeezed into the crowd and reached near the kid with trembling hands to ascultate him, his heart was still beating.We immediately intubated him and shifted him to acute medical care icu.Our critical team was lucky enough to find some iv access and IV fluids, ionotropes were started instantly.

After stabilizing the child i came to PICU. The same tribals have destroyed everything, the beds were lying here and there,chairs were broken, iv stands were dislodged and thrown,glass doors were banged and smashed to the pieces. I told them their child was still alive and had cardiac arrhythmias which was a known complication with the pottasium disturbances in the body.We have counselled them frequently regarding this complication and poor recovery from such illness.They were well aware that child will succumb one or the other day. Still so much havoc...so much destruction...we were getting returns of treating that child free of cost on the humanitarian grounds for many months now.

Police came and booked a few of those tribal people to create a ruckus and took them into the custody.The ladies started crying and pleading to release them. "It was some emotional outbreak and we knew it was totally wrong, please release our men"they started requesting. We can release them but who will pay for all the breakages? Just a single sorry or repenting later can't compensate the huge losses.Our hospital staff started clearing the glasses, all broken things were sent for the repair.I counselled the tribal people and was walking through the hospital lobby when i heard the ambulance siren. It was from the same tribal land. A lady in active labour pains was brought with obstructed labour by our field worker. She was almost on the verge of giving up, totally exhausted dehydrated and drained. Looking at the destruction and havoc created by their own tribal people hospital reception people were refusing to take her. But lives of two was under stake and i couldn't see her dying. We shifted her to emergency OT and operated her. She gave birth to a beautiful angel.There was this sudden happiness and joyous vibes in the Tanda.

They now understood the difference clearly. Although they have smashed and crashed the things and destroyed the hospital, the same doctors helped their people in their tough times.They came in my room and started crying and pleading to forgive them.They were short of words for the way we saved their woman and child. New day had started, sun was rising and making environment more positive. It was long, scary night.Few days later the matter was resolved, local heads and state minister got involved into the issues and compensated for the losses.The tribals in the jails were released.Here both the baby and mother were healthy and ready for discharge. The child with Giettlemans syndrome on ventilator was also stable and fit to go home now although his disease was incurable.We put them all in the ambulance, our field workers were ready to drive them off to their Tanda in the deep forest. All the tribals gathered near my OPD and started bowing together. They hailed my name and invited me for their local function which they have organised to rectify their mistake and to celebrate the arrival of little one. This was the first battle which these tribals have lost in eons of years. But these Lost Tribals looked so happy and elated. Sometimes to loose is the route to happiness.Lost Tribals were waving me bye peeping out from the window and some sitting on the roof of the tempo. I could see their colourful feathers waving in the air.This Loss was their ultimate win.They all were Baazigars to me... Haar ke jitne wale baazigars.Their Loss was their biggest victory ever....!!

* * *

CHAPTER 20

100 DAYS BABY

: My CUG number started beeping continuously tearing the tranquility of the serene night. I got up suddenly from my deep sleep with a jerk and knew it was a dire emergency.Same telephonic ringtones sounds differently on the different occasions.Is it telephonic telepathy that we get aware of emergencies or cold cases from the phone buzz? Only our heart and conscience knows.I drove wildly through the empty streets at the early wee hours.Clock banged 2am past.Doctors cannot run on the clock basis.Emergency doesn't comes by seeing time.Our days becomes night and night becomes day depending on the patients condition.And we tune our bodies to this biological clock rather than inanimate ones. That's why I say Doctor's profession cannot be compared to anyone. We are born to save lives...!!

I reached the NICU almost fleeting the automatic entrance.In the slightest glance i could see the young, educated man standing near the door.His insecurities and worries sensing in the air.A small extremely tiny primie weighing hardly 690gms was lying listlessly in the incubator fighting for life.Hardly could move, hardly could breath,pale, cold,shocky...Such a tiny life struggling hard to survive.Immediately I intubated, instilled surfactant protein directly in the lungs which would help immature lungs to open up and then connected the baby to the ventilator.Inserted a central line, started fluids, BP maintaining medicines, antibiotics to protect the baby from the infections.The umbrella of medical management were started to keep this chotu alive.Our heroic events continues when the entire world enjoys the sugary sleep. After an hour or two of dedicated efforts i managed to stabilize the baby. Baby's father was anxiously waiting for me to update him.He came in the counselling room slightly limping dragging his right leg.Young, tall, very handsome man who spoke softly and listened carefully to understand what his baby's actual problem was.Mother had bad obstetric history with multiple abortions, obestity, had high Bp and raised sugars.She had spontaneous delivery and baby was born with extreme prematurity at 26weeks. I explained father about the prematurity related complications, risks, outcomes, survival chances and short and long term prognosis.Journey was too far and too long with no guaranted outcomes.Really life is unpredictable at every stage.Yet parents were ready to put everything at stake for their baby.

We started putting our efforts at war foot.Doing every possible thing to save this miniature creature which God has sent our way.Such cases are real challenge for we doctors as every new day bring new complications in them and new challenges to us.The baby slowly showed improvement as his activity, perfusion got better. We started to feed this baby slowly with tube.Daily upgrading the amount of feeds as he tolerated. Both the parents religiously attending the baby and doing their every possible bit they can.We were daily tracking the baby's progress closely. Days were passing,time flying and baby was by now one and a half month old.Baby was growing, tolerating full tube feeds,gaining weight.But lung remained immature and was constantly requiring the ventilatory support.We tried our level best, gave trials to wean the baby off from the ventilator but the moment we would remove the tube, baby used to turn blue, desaturate within half an hour and we used to put the baby back on the ventilator.

Parents kept on spending their time, energy, money in the hope that one day they could take their baby home and we were doing our best with a hope to give their precious baby in their laps.True...hope is the only thing which keeps us going.We were trying hard using every possible medical excellence to wean the baby off the ventilator.But sometimes the one above us have different cards to play.And only HE knows our Mastercard.Many a times despite the best efforts lungs doesn't mature well and the damage leads to permanent oxygen dependancy in these babies what we call it as bronchopulmonary dysplasia (BPD) in the medical terms or simply the chronic lung disease.Some babies are lucky enough to get out of the oxygen support or atleast go home on oxygen therapy.But some unfortunate one's like this baby becomes permanently ventilator dependant.

We used all our medical knowledge, used every possible medicine, researched new articles for any new treatment modalities but the baby could not be taken off the machine.Parents were tough and determined and the tiny warrior kept fighting for his every single breath every minute of his life.His sparkling eyes spoke volumes about his will to be alive. We extubated this baby 14 times, everytime with a hope that baby will sustain but for our dismay had to reintubate and put back the baby on ventilator all these 14 times. This is the longest number of intubations and reventilation done by me in my entire career.This case was a real challenge....! Looking at the alert baby gaining weight we struggled hard for his recovery but yet the lungs did not respond.

Every night both parents used to come and sit whole night praying to the Almighty God reciting verses.Their arrival in the Nicu marked exact 10pm in the clock and they spent n numbers of nights beside their ailing baby talking to him to get cured fast.Months went by and every month mother used to paste a paper on the cradle which read "Happy one month my boy...Happy two months my boy! Mother was overweight, heavy lady with chronic diabetes,father had weakness in his right upper limb and right leg post hemiparesis, unable to walk properly but still their physical limitations did not deter their courage and solidarity towards their sick baby.Each and every member in the Nicu including doctors, sisters, aayas, other baby's parents were praying continuously to their respective gods for the well being of this baby.But God had other plans and baby developed severe BPD requiring high settings on the ventilator.We kept on counselling the parents regarding the condition daily and told them it was almost not possible for the baby to survive without ventilator.Still parents continued their efforts without giving up.Parent's love is really unconditional.Nothing in the world can ever replace the parent's love and care for their child.It stems from the heart and it stays eternal..!

Like a regular morning parents came to the Nicu.Mother took out a new dress from her bag,Wore it to the baby,decorated the cradle with the balloons and pasted the note " Happy 100 day's my boy...Thanks for making us the proud parents..!" Tears started rolling heavily on their cheeks, by now they knew the fact that the baby won't survive but they were still proud of their fighter baby who gave them immense happiness of parenthood.This joy is the most precious one which cannot be bought with any money,it cannot be measured but only treasured! These emotions can only be felt and can't be spoken nor expressed.

The baby started having gasping respirations,the light in his eyes started dimming.The heart started missing its beats.Baby turned pale and clammy.We started our resuscitation measures.But time and tide waits for no one.Finally the journey of hundred days came to the halt. Suddenly the dynamic atmosphere of our Nicu was standstill.Inconsolable cries of the parents were putting the invisible cracks in the walls but permanent imprints in our hearts.

Medical science has its own limitations. Despite our wishes and efforts,'HE' keeps ultimate results in his hands.That's why we are humans and HE is the supreme power. With a heavy heart and flowing eyes we bid farewell to our little special guest who stayed the longest with us.Only we know the pain of losing these little warriors as the time binds us together as a family despite their caste, creed,religion,age and the sex.Sometimes the very presence of someone becomes the reason of someone's smile and someone's life. I kept staring into blank, towards the empty cradle of that baby.

"100 days in the Nicu...Thank you for making us feel special by choosing us to be your parents." Last words spoken to the baby by his mother kept echoing in my ears. Really some patients leaves a really strong and permanent impact on our minds.Two years later I got a mail from these parents.curiously I opened the mail which read

"Hundred days of our newborn today..Feels like our boy came back to us.Thank you for all your efforts and love showered. We keep you all in our prayers daily and wanted to share this joy with you all.Love from Emirates."Photo of the newborn was attached with it.It just flashed me of our 100 days baby.He looked exactly the same.My happiness knew no bounds.My mind was in their thoughts.And my hands typed "Thank you so much... Bas Duaon mein yaad Rakhna..!"

* * *

CHAPTER 21

RAB NE BANA DI JODI

Sometimes I feel Life is like the Alibaba's cave...full of history, full of mystries,sometimes dark, sometimes bright and sometimes happy.Everyone you meet here is predestined.Some people meet you to give you the beautiful memories for life and some crosses your path to teach you lessons for life and this one incidence surely made me believe in this.So just remember when Life throws lemons at you make the Lemonade and enjoy it.!!

It was the sunny morning of the early summer.Listening to the morning melodies I drove hurridely through bumpy Hyderabad roads to reach my hospital.Smiling at the gateman and accepting morning wishes from security and ICU staff i entered the Nicu only to greet a small, fragile, very low birth baby staring at me with his wide eyes from his little cradle."Hello little one how are you doing?" I cheered him with a smile.Having difficulty in breathing baby was kept on high flow oxygen, parenteral nutrition,antibiotics and other treatment to support his life.I gave the treatment orders, instructions to the nursing staff, finished my rounds and settled on my counselling chair to talk with the parents to brief them about their ailing kid.This time is tough as you need to adress each and every query of the anxious faces, empathise them and build up their morale and courage.Many a times these times unfolds many unsung stories... Like how it unfolded in this journey.I met this father of this small premie baby unwinding his story.Good morning mam, how is my baby? asked the father in a worried tone.Don't worry,your baby is brave he will improve.I spoke encouragingly. Please do the best possible mam, I don't want my baby to suffer like us.His voice trembled and eyes moistened.We both husband and wife had bad marriages earlier. This is second marriage for both of us.My current wife had abusive marriage, her previous husband was drunkard, used to beat her up often.

Fed up of his physical and mental torture she ran out of his home.Later we met through our families and got married.This baby we had late in our life but I'm happy we have this little bundle of joy to look forward now.His mother had high BP in pregnancy,was on the verge of throwing a fit so have to undergo emergency caesarean madam.Please do save my baby.We have gone through a lot whole life,at least this baby should have a good life.His agonies flowed in his talks and thoughts.Being Parents is really tough..! I assured him about his baby's safety and well being. Seeing all this for a while I thought really the life in the country like ours is so variable and so difficult at times. So many kind of people, different nature, different experiences, everyone fighting their own battles.Every relationship is complex and being non judgemental is truly a tough job.

Eventually this baby improved, started accepting feeds well.Then we called this mother to handle the baby.An elderly mother in her early 40's walked hesitantly in our Nicu.A total village lady, claded in an old saree, big red bindi, handful of green bangles,oily hairs rolled in a messy bun. She stood looking anxious, nervous, hesitant all in one all at a time. I counselled her how to take care of her baby and how to nurse him.Our trained Nicu sisters did their job well and in no time this village woman looked confident and bright.Few days later she was trained in the feeding and we could discharged the baby safely.I gave her instructions to keep the baby warm, feed on time and to come for regular follow ups."Madam you not only saved my baby's life but saved mine too."Coming here to this ICU looking at you I realised how different life is.Squeezed in a muddy abusive life, getting beaten up by my previous husband daily I didn't knew how life looked.But coming here my outlook changed.I now know Life is bigger and can be made better.This second chance in my life with my this good samaritian husband is God's gift to me and I don't want to miss or waste it she told me smilingly as she left the hospital beaming.That day after so many days I could see some different twinkle in her eyes as if they were smiling stars in a dark scary night.

May I come in madam, familiar voice strucked in my opd after few months.I could see a lady carrying a baby in her arms smiling at me.Seetamma is that you?

I literally was taken aback.Total transformation of a village lady into a metro woman.She was wearing a salwar kameez, neatly dressed hair, presentable look with a purse hanging on her shoulder.

I couldn't believe she was the same lady whom i saw a few months ago coming with total make over.Yes mam, she is Seetamma only.She got so much inspired here that she changed herself. I too motivated her and helped her to become her better version said her husband following her.I was so happy to see the kid doing so well.But Seetamma's confidence,her positive attitude,her new outlook towards life, stronger self impressed me more. Yes we don't know what life will serve us in our plates.To accept the situation, to hold on, to move ahead and to grow is what is important in life.Many difficulties will come in everyone's life but to face the challenges with great valour and courage is the most important thing.This couple taught me when life has bad chapters just don't give up but just turn the page, we never know what's there on the flip side.May be happiness and joys in abundance.....

They kept following me on a regular basis.Baby is growing well.Couple are enjoying their second innings.They have overcome their past blues and have accepted the new good life.Suddenly after many months the same father entered my opd with a big smile and a special invitation.Madam Seetamma is pregnant with our second child.Please come for a small get together we have arranged.He handed me the address of a posh restaurant in the city where he was working as stewart.Sure I said, his beaming face became more bright.Thank you madam for showing us silver lining for our cloudy life! He left with great joy.Looking out through my favorite French window I just thought yeah Jodi's are truly made in the heaven. If you get the right partner your life is heaven or else a rutt.And this jodi was really one of it's kind. Rab ne banayi jodi....Sometimes Miracles do happen in life.Like this one. One need to just accept and appreciate it..!!

* * *

CHAPTER 22
FLYING ANGELS

I always say being a doctor we live hundreds of lives in one and expirence rainbow of emotions with each of our patient! Life,death,sorrows,grief,stress and then there comes that billion dollar smile of saving the life,inner peace and satisfaction of the noble deed! Indeed medical life is all the way different.People work,people do jobs but we are the Life savers.Yet along with our efforts there is this divine power guiding us and empowering us all the time helping us out in all our endeavours.And then there are these flying angels around us working behind the scenes and doing more sacred deed than what we do. No words can describe their worth and any appreciation is less for the work they do.Yes they are all walking talking human beings like us yet they are the Angels and knighthoods in the shining armour!!

It was around 4am in the early morning when this case came to us.A five day old baby getting treated for high jaundice was being referred from the peripheral hospital as the baby has thrown fits.My mobile beep interrupted my deep sleep and my hand reflexly went to my phone.We as a doctor are so used to our mobile ringtone that even amidst of my deepest sleep cycle I recive call at second ring.Really our profession teach us many things!

Mam baby is sick,dull and had fits.We have loaded with a drug to control fits. Jaundice is high so have started the baby on intensive phototherapy lights.My neonatal fellow on duty was updating me the case scenario.I instructed him few more things to stream line the treatment part.My mental mapping alarmed me that I have to reach hospital sooner to tackle this case.I reached the hospital rather early as I anticipated baby was very sick with high jaundice.Report reading 32,requiring urgent blood exchange.Mother's and baby's blood groups were incompatible,mother being Rh negative and baby Rh positive.Dct was strongly positive.This is the setting where jaundice rises too rapidly,reaches the brain making the baby to throw fits and even causing permanent brain damage leaving the blood exchange transfusion only choice to save baby's life!

We immediately intubated the baby and connected her to the ventilator.Central line was placed through the umbilical route for blood exchange and now we had to arrange for the blood.It was a major task to find negative blood group as it's very rare group to find and not easily available.I personally called almost 35 blood banks to find the required blood but was unfruitful.We checked the blood groups of baby's relatives but those were also different. Everyone was trying their level best to arrange the blood but every effort was going in vain. It was becoming extremely difficult to get a negative group for exchange transfusion.And then i thought to try some other ways to get blood and what else could be more powerful than social media these days. I circulated the message in my friends group,Facebook etc thinking at least it may be of some use.And to my surprise i started getting instant responses from the people whom I never knew,whom I have never met.They started working for us,circulating the message and spreading the word. My friend's friends,their distant relatives,people working for social cause all started working together for one Nobel cause of saving life without knowing the name,religion,caste,creed,age or sex just to lend a helping hand! Within an hour Mr Shitanshu Gupta arranged donor for us.I never met him nor did I knew him but a single message of blood requirement was enough for them to get started.We circulated message in my Marathi Doctors group in Hyderabad and one of my medico colleague Dr Shreyas a surgeon by profession again whom i haven't seen nor met came straight out of his OT,travelled more than 25 Kms and donated blood for this unknown kid. Next donor was young college going engineering student merely 24-25 years old.He also travelled more than 30 Kms and did his very first blood donation.I was amazed and astonished by this kind of instant response.Never in my wildest dreams I ever thought there would be these kind of angels who fly high from the far away places to help selflessly.

Within two-three hours two donors donated blood,processing done and we were able to do exchange transfusion for our this sick baby.Shitanshu was in constant touch asking about baby's progress and if more blood was required to be arranged.He even alerted his friends who posted the requirement in other groups and to my astonishment I recieved many calls and messages of the people willing to help.There were many doctors especially a lady doctor who herself called and told she was of negative blood group and was ready to donate. Then there was Dr Chetan Mundada our previous pediatric consultant and the gem of the person who called to inform us that he was also O negative and would donate the blood if required.In today's era where corrupt media and sold politicos keep tarnishing, blaming doctors, people like Dr Chetan,Dr Shreyas and Mr Shitanshu stands tall.

How many of we doctors or even patient's relatives donate blood without a second thought.Here all these people who helped us were totally unknown.They came they helped and left without creating a buzz or without expecting a single penny.People say they believe in God..aren't these kind of people the God of current era? So helpful and yet so selfless.These qualities are really rare and because of such people my faith in humanity and goodness of people is still unstirred ! These kind of people are good Samaritans and knighthoods in the shining Armours! Many people boast of the social service they do and then there are these kind of people who keep working without making noise collecting the brownie points of their good deeds.

Don't know how to thank these people,don't know what words would be enough for their appreciation but I realised one thing we strive hard to save life within four walls of our hospital and then there are these people who keep helping us behind the scene to make our endeavours successful.I will be always grateful for all these people who helped us instantly to save the baby's life.You guys are real hero's and the gem of the people which world needs more. I never knew social media would be so powerful and impactful.All over the night I was thinking that World is full of miracles.This baby coming to our unit,we requiring blood of rare group,it's non availability in all the blood banks and then arrival of all these super heroes on time and helping the baby out.Everything was miraculous.Does the universe wanted to retain my faith in humanity and brotherhood by showing such people? I really don't know.That's why I say miracles do happen and yes definitely they do!!!!

* * *

CHAPTER 23

A BIG STORY OF BIG STOMACH

Titoo..titoo...titooo...ambulance siren came ringing aloud.Emergency case to the Nicu,call banged on the speaker from the reception.Antenas of our mind stood erect and hands started working even more faster.More rapid were my thoughts mental mapping for the treatment of the receiving baby.The doors of lift were opened hurriedly,the sound of transport incubator gave us the news of baby's arrival.Our warmers were on,prewarmed towels,gloves,suction catheters,intubation instruments and all the essential drugs were ready on the crash trolley neatly arranged. Oxgen flow meters were on with ventilator by the side. The entire setting was arranged within fraction of second as we recived the small tiny baby fighting to breath in the warmer. Preterm of 26-27 weeks weighing hardly 1 kg trying his best to keep his respiration going on.

These babies are the true fighters.I immediately intubated the baby and put him on to the ventilator. Central line was put and parenteral nutrition started,basic things needed for the micro primis survival.Ventilator assured his breathing and TPN assured nutrition.Investigations were sent and then my eyes caught the person standing in a corner of our counselling room with newly made baby's case sheet in his hand.Are you with the baby? my gentle question. Yes madam i'm baby's uncle,please save this child.Mother is also very serious she has lost lots and lots of blood before the delivery.APH we call it as in the medical language. Ante-partum hemorrhage the most unfortunate event for the pregnant lady.(and a dire emergency for the gynaecologists).She had severe complications and is on ventilator so please save this baby.The uncle lost his emotions in the tears which ran down continuously on his cheeks.I spoke to him empathetically and ensured him to do our level best while explaining him the complications of prematurity and very low birth weight babies.His eyes were searching hopes in me.Being a doctor we know their emotions but to tell the fact is our duty.

sometimes facts are more teary than the emotions! Baby was sick,laboratory reports were bad with initial platelets being very low.We started the baby on the antibiotics and ionotropic support.After the intial stabilization small amount of feeds were started through the nasogastric tube and to our dismay on the 3rd day baby's abdomen bloated and was very tense.We were disheartened as it's one more dreaded complication - Necrotising enterocolitis where baby is unable to digest milk and in the background of infection it leads to intestinal swelling and inflammation.It adds on to the complication for treatment.Next few days we were struggling to stabilize the baby.

Abdomen was distended but to our surprize baby was passing motion.Baby remained listless on the ventilator with stomach remained bloated.Pediatric surgeon was called in and i was frantically behind him to operate on this baby to relive the distention as keeping the baby in such condition would have damaged the intestines further. Xrays of abdomen showed dilated loops but the expirenced eyes of our Pediatric Surgeon were not convinced to operate.He told us to continue the medical management further.Whole night i was thinking about the baby.General parameters were improving,Septic screen showed improving platelets,baby was passing motion yet abdomen was distended.What was this mystery behind his bloated and distended abdomen? Mystery of his big stomach? I kept on thinking and thinking and something striked my mind like a lightening flash as if i got the answer.Next day i ordered for the thyroid profile of this baby and to our despair baby's TSH was very very very high(above 150).It was the eureka moment for us as we cracked the case but nonetheless for the baby.We spoke to the pediatric endocrinologist and without losing a single minute we started the baby on thyroid supplement and what a miracle...three days down the lane baby's abdominal swelling and distention decreased; abdomen became soft. Baby was started on feeds and was upgraded to full feeds shortly. Baby was extubated, put on high flow oxygen and then gradually weaned to the room air within few days.Thyroid nuclear scan done was suggestive of thyroid dyshormonogenesis..i.e.thyroid hormones werent formed properly.

Thyroid supplement was increased as TSH remained high. To add on the baby developed severe jaundice involving liver.Anti cholestatic measures were started. Baby kept fighting all odds although being diagnosed with a hole in heart(moderate ASD).Baby kept his fighting spirit high to improve slowly and steadily. Meanwhile mother also improved and came in for baby's care. Baby kept improving steadily day by day,started accepting oral feeds and later was discharged with consistent weight gain.T4 levels normalised with TSH although being little on the higher side which later normalized.

After one and a half month of turmulous and stormy neonatal course we were happy to discharge the baby in stable condition.I kept on thinking on this case for a long time before penning it down. I have seen many of us don't even give a thought for thyroid testing . Although many babies are screened normal, one among them like this can come out as a bolt from the blue. It's very neccesary to diagnose hypothyroidism at the earliest and to start the treatment early as the only small step of thyroid supplement can save the babie's brain and prevent mental retardation.So guys the message from this post is not to forget to check thyroid levels in all the babies born term/ preterm,normal weight/ low birth weight as one single check can save the life. Congenital hypothyroidism can present in various ways and NEC like picture can be it's one presentation in newborn period. It was miraculous that we could diagnose it as early as in the first week of life and started it's treatment at the earliest.Finally the mystery of big stomach was solved in a big way! Indeed a story to remember!!

* * *

CHAPTER 24
BILLION DOLLAR LIFE

"Code blue in casualty"there was an emergency announcement from the reception. I hurriedly fleeted to the casualty from the middle of my lunch. My other team mates also joined me shortly. Code blue is for sudden cardiac arrest and is an extremely urgent scenario to be attended.Our doctor on duty in OPD has already started initial rescucitation measure and have kept the life support system ready. I saw a young girl of 8-9 years lying listless on the bed throwing multiple seizures and was almost gasping. Being trained in the emergency management we instantly did role allotment and our emergency minds were at work. Flock of nurses came for help. IV lines were secured,Fluid boluses were given,Medicines to raise BP were started and the drugs to control the fits were initiated.Airways were taken care of and the child was intubated and ventilated. After 45 minutes of heroic events child was stabilsed. I told further line of management to my juniors and walked to meet the parents.

How is my child Doctor? Emotional Father could barely ask.He looked like a simple village man in a dhoti and pancha, like a priest in the temple.Hello I'm your baby's Doctor. Your child is having high grade fever,her BP is low and she's throwing multiple fits.We have started her on all the needed treatment.Her condition is critical and she is on life support system.But be positive and just keep praying.We will do our best i tried consoling the parents.I could see the mother sobbing relentlessly in a corner. Her running eyes raised thousands of questions behind her silent face. By the way when did it all started I asked empathetically to know the background history although it was looking like a case of viral encephalitis to me.

Madam I work as a priest in the Shiva temple. She is our only child born after 12 years of marriage.We have done lots of pujas,Vrathas,fastings after which god gifted us with this beautiful child.She is always a topper in her school and has beautiful voice.She is well known for reciting beautiful Shiva bhakti geets and the bhajans.For the past one week she is having high grade fever and she wasn't eating anything.We took her to our village doctor for the treatment.But from today morning she started having fits so we rushed here finally...father broke into tears.Save her at any cost Madam...She is my only reason to live.My in-laws wanted me to divorce my husband as I couldn't give them a grand child.I did Sola-Somvaar vratha to Lord mahadev and he gifted me this baby.Please save her crying mother pleaded.Child was critical and situation was tough.Being a treating doctor I was the only ray of hope for them.We will try our level best"Trust Him, We treat, HE cures.."! I said assuringly.

We shifted the child to the ICU.Her all IV access were exhausted and she required central line for multiple drips.Internal jugular was set in.she was treated in full force.After 5 days of her battle with the wild notorious virus we could stabilise her and our treatment started showing results.Her sensorium improved and by now she was fighting on the ventilator.We did a planned extubation. She got better days after days and was discharged in the stable condition.Intermittently father used to call and inform us about her well being. We visited the Shiva temple on one of the Sravan somvaar. Some times God has destined to meet some people to gain some good will.

Time flew and we were busy in our daily routine. And one fine day I saw the same priest carrying her daughter in his arms in full panic mode. He was drenching in the sweat when the child lied listless in his arms.I got up from my chair in a moment to examine her.She was unresponsive and pale.Pulses were feeble, she was in shock. Her breathing was feeble.What happened to her I asked the father worriedly. She fell down from a tree while playing madam.One of the branch had fallen on her chest and she suddenly became unconscious father told in trembling voice.

We too trembled as we put her on oxygen and started iv fluids.Her chest wasn't rising. We took an emergency bed side chest xray.Her half of the chest was completely hazy,opposite lung was compressed,heart was shifted to the opposite side. Signs of hydropneumothorax (means collection of air and the fluid in the chest). We immediately intubated her,Secured her breathing and in the brisk of time I inserted a chest tube. It's called Intercoastal drainage tube which drains air and fluid from the chest and helps the lungs to expand. But to our surprise it was pool of blood seeping forcefully from the chest tube. It was just like fresh blood coming out from the open tap.We arranged for the blood instantly.Mean while we started pushing IV fluids to maintain her circulation and BP. We were in the dilemma from where did this sea of blood is pouring? Then my thinking mind gave me a clue. I hurriedly connected the ultrasound machine and examined her.One of her major artery was torn and hence she was bleeding profusely. I was really worried by now as it was a dire emergency to suture the torn vessel at the earliest to stop the bleeding and there was no other go.We have literally pumped pints and pints of blood.She was bleeding like a running tap from her chest and we were literally pumping the blood in an attempt to keep her alive. It was the game of hide and seek between the life and death!

Cardiothoracic surgeon was called in on the emergency basis and Emergency OT was scheduled.We all doctors with our team of nurses, Surgeon and the entire OT staff were battling in the operation theatre forgetting our hunger cramps and our thirst. Our minds knew only one job.. to work tirelessly to save the life.We were standing continuously with our hands working relentlessly doing everything we knew and helping the surgeon to find out the tear so he can suture it . Finally the artery was sutured and bleeding stopped.It was already early morning by then.Packs and packs of blood was transfused and almost many of our doctors, nursing staff on the duty have donated their blood to save this young life.It was morning 4am when we walked out of the OT. We shifted her back to the ICU on the ventilator.Fluids and ionotropes were titrated to control her BP and to maintain circulation.It was all dark and silent outside.Only the sound of beeping ventilator and pulseoximeter moniters breached the serene peace and silence.

We collapsed in the chairs in the canteen as we sipped on the hot coffee,the most needed break in the past 24 hrs.We were the mute spectators of this horrendous war between life and death. Our bodies were worned out but heart was at bliss as we could save this life at last. What a night..no..no it was a night mare!.

Madam can we come in? Soft voice broke our thinking process. We were in the temple all night praying to God for the safety of my child.God has acted through you people to save our girl.We will never forget this moment till our last breath as she is our precious daughter.. parents spoke gratitudely. They put Prasad of Lord Shiva on my palm.Tears rushed on their cheeks and the child's mother was speechless.Her sparkling eyes spoke volumes of gratitude. She is all fine now,we will extubate her in the next 24 Hours and send her home in next 4-5 days probably I updated them. She is God gifted so Lord Shiva has done the miracle of tiding this crisis and saving her life.A peaceful smile spread on their face.True...hard work,dedication and selfless intentions works miracles! This case was one of its kind which was permanently etched to my mind as we really swimmed across the ocean of blood and had reached the shore safely.This was a billion dollar life indeed!

* * *

CHAPTER 25

NAVADURGA OF GENERATION X

Strolling towards my evening opd, amongst many parents waiting with their tiny tots to consult me i couldn't miss those dull yet tenacious eyes smiling at me.A faint smile lingered on my face brightening up my evening.Yeah some patients of yours bring that unknown smile to your face every time you see them.

On her turn she came inside with a baby grown now as close to 9 months.Smiling carefree he was enjoying the varieties of things spread on my table.Then Geeta did you find any name for your boy or not yet ? My usual question in every month's consultation for her followed by her familiar answer" No mam, his father is still searching the name, he is too busy with his work.

From the early trimester, i see this lady coming alone for the hospital visits, her husband being professor in some remote college was too busy shuttling between home and work and was too busy to accompany her for her antenatal check ups. It was her second child and this baby was detected with fetal anemia in the early pregnancy due to blood group mismatch.Mother being Rh Negative and baby Rh Positive, it's very much likely that second born and thereafter babies born may develop severe anemia (low Hb) in fetal life and also may develop early onset severe jaundice.

We were following her closely as her Mom(multiples of median) on graphs were crossing the danger zone suggesting the baby is getting anemic inside the mother's womb requiring intrauterine blood transfusions. We counselled her that we need to transfuse blood to the baby directly in the mothers womb or else baby might develop complications and may have heart failure.Listening to this her fragile face became more dull,eyes looked more pale but her mind did not deter.

Mam, you go ahead and do whatever is needed for my baby's health.Im ready to tolerate all the hassles but my baby should be safe she said assertively.We told her to call her husband but as usual he was too busy to attend her or accompany her.She herself did visits to the blood banks,we helped her out with all other formalities and called her husband during the procedure.He just came like a guest lecturer in his college, did his job of signing the consent form, waited till the procedure was over and left. But this lady didn't had any qualms,nor queries,nor complaints about her husband.Mam he is too stressed out traveling daily from one city to other for his job.I don't want to trouble him more with these all additional work.I was there in USA for 3 years for my Masters in Economics.My in laws were not much in favour of me going abroad for my higher studies.They wanted me to be here and attend my household duties as a good daughter in law but my passion,my dreams did not allow me to be in the kitchen so i took my entire responsibility, got student Visa, got scholarship in USA, did my masters and returned back to my Motherland with much pride she told her story with a smile.This time i could see that little twinkles in her eyes making them more shiny and bright!!

Behind such a simple,ordinary looking housewife wrapped

in a simple worn out cotton churidar was a well read,well travelled and well educated woman.No doubt she was shouldering all responsibility of her baby alone.I was much more in awe of her now after knowing her story.Indian Women are really strong.They do face all the life's challenges, work so hard and stand rock steady alone fighting life's all odd.We did intrauterine fetal blood transfusions thrice for her baby.Everytime she used to come, listen patiently to all our advice, do all the arrangements and formalities for the procedure promptly.No many questions,no anxiety but only full trust on us with just one line at end "Do whatever is required Madam, but my baby should be safe".Yeah it should be i used to answer with a smile back to her.And this went on for a while.

And then after 36 weeks she delivered her second baby boy albeit growth retarded weighing 2kgs but all hale and hearty. Because of our antenatal well controlled treatment baby did not develop much jaundice nor required any more blood transfusions later.We were happy that all the trouble we took in counselling the patient and their attenders, vigilant monitoring her through out the pregnancy, arranging for negative blood group which rare and quiet difficult to procure and carrying over the very tedious process of fetal transfusion not once but thrice. Everything we did,we toiled was fallen in proper place. And when we the Doctors see such babies coming out hale and hearty that pleasure is just immeasurable!

Like a dotting mother she took all the possible care of her baby.Every visit postnatally for vaccines and the follow ups showed baby's excellent growth and development.Near about past 9 months i was seeing her all alone attending my opds, maintaining all the records,taking care of immunization, baby diet, medications and almost everything.Every month i used to ask her "Alone this time too? And she used to reply calmly "His father is too busy with his work madam."No complaints no qualms.But i used to go frenzy every time with her cool answer.

This time as she entered my consultation room,i read the name on the case paper and it wasn't B/0 Geeta anymore.It was Ekant,i was surprised and beamingly asked her so his father finally got some time to find the name for his baby then? She smiled softly yeah mam he was finding some uncommon name.My elder son's name is Azad as he was born on 15th August and now he is Ekant as he spent most of the time aloof and alone in the Nicu after he was born she told the story behind his name. Oh that's good i said but was surprised to see so much mental and emotional power these Indian women carry with them with so much Alan.She was doing everything alone for her baby from almost early days of her pregnancy without much support from her family or her in laws.Leave about the physical support but not even moral support but still she was so calm composed and determined.Not complaining about anything and anyone but accepting Life gracefully as it comes.

I felt that really she is the Navadurga of today's generation.Generation X what we call as where families are nuclear and relations are namesake.She was simple looking Navadurga but full of power.Power to walk down life alone with full courage, power to wither life's all odd alone but still standing here with a smiling face just looking forward and making everything possible for her baby's laughter. And then i realised that's the power of being a mother going to any extent in true sense for her baby's well being.I could see her playing carefree with her naughty baby boy.His loud innocent smile was echoing in my room.We fondly call him Tiger madam she chirped happily hugging her baby.Yeah and "You are the tigress embracing your life alone courageously " i said patting her back gently.She waved with a faint smile and walked out of my opd. I knew from within a month she will be back again alone with her baby answering to my familiar question saying "His father is too busy shuttling with his work madam and i dont want to trouble him with this additional work." I smiled at her thoughts as i never knew raising a child could be mere an additional work to someone. And such a fierce sole Navadurgas like Geeta stand still taller in this today's World for me.More power to you my girl i whispered to myself.And this is how life goes on. Looking at her i realised its truely said "Those who fly solo have the toughest wings"...!!

* * *

CHAPTER 26
AFTER THE STORM

It was raining cats and dogs outside,the howling winds were busy smashing the window panes on each other.Thunderous storm and lightning embarked on the nearby panel followed by loud sound turning our ears momentarily deaf.We haven't seen the light yet.. it's been more than 3 days now we were stucked in our hospital room.Clouds were bursting,rains were pouring and we were hit by the massive floods.The roads and ditches were full of water and the water level was rising day by day.

Transportation was toppled and people have migrated to higher places trying to save their lives.People were more humanitarian, accommodating each other in their houses and sharing their food.Survival was the only aim here.Floods were heavy and people suffered a lot.Our hospital was full with patients suffering from fever,chills, loose motions, malaria ,dengue and leptospira on rise.Beds and beds were getting full and now it was time to put matress in between two cots and treat the patient.It was the testing times for doctors as well.There cannot be anything higher in front of God's wish and natures will! We humans at times feel so helpless! Life has come to a complete halt.

It was my 3rd on call day.Our other colleagues were stucked in their homes and couldn't commute because of heavy floods.We at hospital were staying in doctors room and working day and night to help people survive.Rescue force was getting flocks and flocks of people from various location entrapped in water and we were trying to bring their physical as well as mental well being back." Mam one lady is in labour, she will deliver now we want you here".i got a call from the Labour room in charge sister.Yes i will be there at the next moment,i assured her.I gave the treatment order for my patients in the emergency room who has survived near drowning state in flood waters and turned back to the labour room.

Baby delivered and he was healthy 3 kg's boy.He looked around and gave a hearty cry.His twinkling eyes brought feeling of joy in that serious damp weather.We wrapped him in the warm towel after routine care and handed him to his mother for feeding.Normal delivery and Normal Mother and baby was surely a bliss in these hard times.We sent them home the very next day as they stayed in the neighbourhood. On the 4th day again granny brought the baby wrapped in the torn saree cloth.Please check him urgently madam she said in a panicky mode.I opened the cloth just to find baby lying dull and groaning.Ohh my god what happened to him..our nicu nurse exclaimed as she could sense his condition.He is not drinking milk properly since yesterday madam, his mother is also sick, getting fever since 2nd day of delivery. She is getting iv fluids daily in the emergency room as there are no beds to admit her so they told her to come daily and get treated on the OPD basis grandmother told in the helpless tone. Yeah beds were full and priority was given to sick and the critical patients for admission. I took the baby inside the nicu and recorded his temperature.He was febrile, dehydrated and had developed jaundice.Weight loss of 17% was more as the mother was unable to feed the baby. We immediately started him on the treatment.Measures were taken to control fever,IV fluid was started to correct dehydration,antibiotics were started and baby was kept under phototherapy for jaundice. After settling this baby i ranged in Emergency room to find out mother's condition. She has got dengue,her NS 1 is positive but otherwise she is clinically stable.Our ER doctor briefed me her condition. For our luck baby's all reports were on the normal side.

Next day baby showed improvement, fever was controlled, jaundice was less and baby was accepting feeds well. We noticed weight gain as well so it was a dehydration fever. We involved the mother in feeding and shifted the baby to the mother side. Next day was uneventful and we prepared both mother baby duo for the discharge coming morning.I came early and did my Nicu rounds.I entered the KMC room with a notion to discharge the baby but as I opened the baby's wrap I could see again the baby groaning. Temperature recorded was 104 f and i could sense the storm coming. I counselled the parents and shifted the baby to nicu. Immediately baby was started on oxygen, ivf ,antibiotics and other supportive measures. Blood tests were sent and reports were traced urgently. And to my dismay reports were too bad indicating baby's critical nature. Platelets have dropped from 2 lakhs to 20,000. Coagulation profile (blood clotting factors) were highly deranged. Baby started deteriorating with increase in breathing difficulty. Baby was pale and in shock. We immediately ventilated the baby, transfused platelets and fresh frozen plasma,BP medicines were hiked up. Additional medicines were started to control the circulatory disturbances.Liver enzymes were highly elevated indicating failing liver. Chest scan and abdominal scan indicated fluid collection. Dengue Ns1 was positive this time yet Dengue antibodies were negative. We were dealing with a rare condition of Congenital Dengue with Dengue Shock syndrome. Baby was critical fighting for life and we had very little hope that baby could survive this acute and critical phase. We have seen children rapidly deteriorating going in ARDS and dying within a span of few hours with severe dengue. But this baby was fighter and so were we. Being in the ICU and working with critical babies we have developed this never say die attitude. I work relentlessly and treat my patients with full dedication irrespective of their end results. Next platelets read 8000 which was too low and baby started showing bit of bleeding tendency by now. Mother, Grand father had given up the hope and our hearts too started sinking.

We transfused multiple units of SDP, Fresh frozen plasma and Prbc. In v/0 life threatening condition we thought of transfusing the baby with iv immunoglobulin which was the last resort and ray of hope but again very costly. Patients were poor and couldn't afford the basic treatment so expecting them to get this exobirantly high rated ivig was not possible. Sometimes somewhere it happens that you could relate to your patients and you feel more humanitarian than doctor. Its important to transfuse ivig, get it started il pay for it i ordered my residents. We give each other some breeze of positivity with these kinds of deeds intermittently. Sometimes we donate our blood in emergency to our patients and sometimes we do monetary help which goes unnoticed. Rather it's kept under wraps because we tend to live as doctors and not God.

Slowly the strong will power of the baby and our hard work paid off and baby started showing signs of improvement.Bp maintained, urine output improved,fluid collection in serous cavities resolved, breathing difficulty was controlled now. Platelets gradually showed improving trend.We weaned off the baby from ventilator to Cpap and then to oxygen and room air in next 4 days.Slowly feeds were started via nasogastric tube and slowly spoon feeds were started. Now the baby looked much better,pink and breathing at ease in room air. Platelets and Coagulation parameters were normal. Liver enzymes were normalised too. Baby survived this stormy course and got the new lease of life.

We handed the baby to mother and she broke into tears." I never thought I will get my baby back madam.we have lost all our hopes. You gave him new life...I will never forget your hardships."She hugged the baby and both cried together.These were tears of joy. Grand father took out his old cloth bag and kept small steel box in my hand. We got sheera in this, Satyanarayan swami prasad madam.We prayed god for his well being and he answered our prayers.We haven't seen God yet but for us you are the living God who brought our baby to life from death bed, he became emotional. I opened his box and took some kesari halwa and distributed rest among my staff. Everyone got their share of blessings from the God for the selfless hardwork and for the noble deed they did. We waved them as they left the ward happily. These moments are really pure bliss.

Rains have stopped by now and sun was peeping from the clouds spreading his warm rays of positivity and hopes. World was slowly getting back on the track.Life after the storm was more valued as it taught us all to fight the life's every odd and this fighter baby taught us never to give up in any situation but rather to keep going with will, vigour and valour. We were happy to diagnose one of the rare case of Congenital Dengue and treat it successfully. Storms inside and outside were more calmer now!!

* * *

CHAPTER 27
A SMALL WONDER

It was mid August time and wednesday night.Clock ranged 2 am, dark night was getting more darker, gush of wind was entering the window disturbing the cool breeze.After a very busy and hectic schedule i was deep asleep in my cosy warm bed.Suddenly the silent night was disturbed by my noisy phone ring.I being too tired picked up phone sluggishly and was barely able to say hello. Really some days are too exhausting!

Hi mam,one preterm baby has got admitted with respiratory distress.I'm sending you her xray,one side of chest is hazy,other side looking too hyperinflated i think its pneumothorax, shall I put an icd? My resident doctor in nicu was asking me impatiently.The word pneumothorax suddenly recharged my brain and i came to my senses as the pneumothorax is a dire Medical emergency in the newborn.Wait let me see the xray once i told and I scrolled my watsapp for the xray picture sent and i was taken aback.The xray looked more of pneumothorax, left side chest was hyper inflated(highly expanded) and right side was hazy but my brain attenea was giving me different signal.No it's not just a plain pneumothorax why the complete chest on right is hazy?? Is it more of contralateral hyperinflation(opposite lung being more expanded) due to the lung pathology on right?? My mind got on to the work.It looked more like Congenital Lung malformation to me.Sometimes our intutions are too strong to ignore.Just get a CT scan chest quick I told my resident.And yes my experienced eyes had got it right it was right sided Complete Agenesis of lung(non development of lung) which indicates by birth baby did not have lung on one side and was struggling for life on only one single lung. It's time to rush, I got up hurriedly and reached the hospital in no time.For any emergency you have to pick up your own sore body and have to get on working as it's the question of life and death. And we doctors are Messiah who save lives many a times at the cost of our own life.

I rushed to the Nicu and met my resident at the door who was shifting the baby from the CT room. I examined baby thoroughly. Many a times one major anamoly is associated with other anomolies involving other organs. Heart,Brain and abdomen were scanned. Everything looked to be placed in position. Heart,liver,stomach all were well placed.Quiet a few times single lung is associated with right sided heart and shuffling of liver and stomach to the opposite side. But this baby didn't have those problems luckily. I ventilated the baby and stabilised the lungs, IV Fluids and other treatment was started. Once I was sure that baby is settled I walked to the counseling room to talk to the attenders. Making attenders/parents to understand about such rare condition is the major task. Convincing them and making them to accept the fact is still harder.

I broke the news to the family in subtle way with empathy.They were shocked and blank as they didn't knew how and what to react.Their face looked worried and full of questions.Only one lung? Will this baby survive with single lung they asked with crying tone,eyes almost full of tears. We have heard of single kidney madam but baby with a single lung? we are hearing it for the first time they were in shock still.Yeah i can understand your anxiety it's very new thing for you but babies with single lung do exist and many a times people with this problem present in adulthood as well. They remain asymptomatic throughout their childhood and are diagnosed coincidently. But few cases are diagnosed at birth who presents early in life with breathing difficulty i was explaining them the complex thing in the easiest possible language. It is very important to keep this baby safe and away from infections as a single episode of infection would decompensate the baby badly..i was trying to stress the gravity of the problem to them.Finally we have kidney transplant even heart transplant system available but lung transplant is still at bay and this is one area in the field of Medicine which is still evolving i cautioned parents so that they can understand the criticality of their baby and how meticulously they should take care of him.

Father was in a state of confusion, relatives started whispering some evil eye might have preyed on her during her pregnancy that's why she delivered such an abnormal baby. She must have done some sin so she got punished in this way.Talks and talks and those were unending. In India still in today's era women are blamed for every single thing. I kept on educating relatives on this condition for days together,showed them literature, photos and videos till the day they came to the terms. Now they weren't fully convinenced but were slowly realising and accepting the things. Mother was depressed and was sobbing continuously why me and why my baby? i did every possible thing,followed every ritual, ate healthy, took good care of my self in whole 9 months, i never had any minor problem in entire course then why i had this kind of baby? Why god gave such a big problem to my baby? She was asking us relentlessly. Yes some why's have no answer. We consoled her and gave her moral support. We took her to the baby cradle and showed her the baby.The little ball of flesh was lying in comfy bed breathing slowly.The gentle touch of baby melted her heart... at the end of the day she was a mother. Natural instinct of acceptance flows through her blood. Now why me? Why my baby and all such questions were irrelevant to her. Seeing her baby alive brought a twinkle in her eyes and now she was all ready to do anything and everything possible to make her baby survive.

Days passed on and on.Slowly baby started showing the signs of improvement. Breathing problem settled,tube feeds were continued. Baby was extubated after 3 days and gradually brought to the room air in a weeks time. Mother visited her baby daily and started handling him.Mother's touch has great healing power. Slowly she was involved in the tube feeds and then baby was discharged when mother was confident enough to handle the baby and to feed her by tube.We were happy that we could send the baby with single lung home. Every week parents kept visiting me for the follow up. Baby was quiet comfortable and was growing well on tube feeds.

But to our dismay at 45 days of life baby came to us with severe distres.The breathing was fast and laboured.Baby was turning blue intermittently.This time baby looked more sick requiring more oxygen.Time to ventilate again.We counselled the parents and ventilated the baby.Xray chest showed bronchiolitis (Viral Pneumonia).Antiviral drugs were started along with empirical antibiotics and other supportive measures.Baby was unable to maintain saturations and required High frequency ventilation.Daily day in and out baby was fighting for each single breath. Only one single existing lung was trying hard to compensate the workload.We all could see that the survival chances were bleak.We kept counseling regarding the guarded prognosis to the parents.Parents obliged to our treatment and respected our words and kept praying whole heartedly.Many a times faith and prayers overpowers the clinical logic and Miracles do happen.After 12 days of dreadful battle for life on High frequency ventilation baby slowly started showing improvement.Breathing difficult was slowly reducing and we could decrease the ventilator settings.Tube feeds were restarted. With good nutrition and good medications baby improved faster and was extubated shortly.Baby was breating on oxygen and tolerating tube feeds.We taught mother to give nebulisation and gave her tips to prevent future infections in her baby. She was working hard day and night for his well being. Baby was now comfortable at room air and we shifted them to room. Both parents were taking good care of the baby and he improved faster and was off oxygen.

I went to their room for my evening rounds.Next day was their discharge. I appreciated the parents for their extraordinary efforts. "It's all your efforts madam,our baby came out of death bed twice because of your hard work and treatment. Without you he wouldn't have seen the light of this day.Parents work hard because it's their baby, but doctors do things selflessly although they do not share any blood relation with their patients.You are really God sent to us"they said in a trembling voice. "We doctors do our duty whole heartedly and give our 200% for every case. It's very heartening to see babies doing good. Doctors give medicine but its parents strong will power which bring back their babies back to life" i told them.

As I entered hospital next day i could see my entire nursing staff in cheerful mood. Ward was decorated with balloons and i could feel birthday vibes in the air. Today we are celebrating birthday of our single lung baby before discharge they chirped happily. Birthday? I said surprisingly. Yeah Mam you gave him new lease of life and we are going home so its his birthday in real sense today father said as he walked with delicious cake in his hand. Never to say we celebrated his birthday with great zeal and zest. And from then on they celebrate his birthday every year in our hospital.It's been 3 years now and baby is doing fine. Really it's well said in marathi "Dev Tari tyala kon mari"..means when the creator is the protector, every person is a survivor! Parents walked happily with their small wonder wrapped in the warm cosy clothes. May this small wonder do wonders in his life I blessed him with a smile and turned to my work of saving many other wonderful lives.

* * *

CHAPTER 28

GULLY BOY

It was a very busy and sunny summer afternoon.After the hectic grand rounds on Thursday i was heading towards the canteen for some refreshing drink when my phone rang just to signal an emergency in the ER.I rushed to emergency room to find out a young boy of 14-15 years gasping for his breaths.His saturation was 70% at room air.Our ER doctor and nursing staff were on their toes to stabilize him.He was breathing heavily and sweating profusely,even with oxygen support his saturation could hardly reach 85%. He was highly febrile with a temperature of 103F.He is very critical and requires to be ventilated immediately,i alerted my team.Within no time crash trolley was pulled, Ambu bag and the mask were ready,all the emergency drugs were loaded and under Rapid Sequence technique intubation was done and he was connected to the ventilator.Fluid boluses were given, IV fluids and BP controlling medications were started and after initial stabilization he was shifted to the ICU.

His fever was recurring and he was not very well responding to the paracetamol and antibiotics.In the ICU our great minds started at work.Blood investigations were sent, Xray Chest was done.Complete blood picture showed high levels of eosinophils, IgE levels were high.Chest xray showed some fluffy shadows.CT Chest confirmed the diagnosis.Yes it was a very rare disease and it was Eosinophilic Pneumonia! Generally this disease has poor outcome and poor prognosis.We started him on steroids, the drug used in high Eosinophilic conditions.Antihistaminics, supportive treatment was continued.Child slowly recovered and was weaned off the ventilator after few days.Now he was breathing at ease and accepting some oral fluids.

Hi Ibrahim how are you feeling now? i asked him in my morning rounds.I'm feeling much better madam, please discharge me by Sunday at any cost he said pleadingly.OK you are doing good, shall discharge you soon.But what's special about Sunday? now don't tell me you are going to play a cricket match at Wankhede stadium i said laughing.Nahi Madam Monday subah jaldi jaana hai shiv ji k mandir...Phool, Belpatri dena rehta hai na logon ko,he said worriedly.Main nahi rahunga toh logon ko phool kahase milenge? I was surprised to hear this.You sell flowers outside shivalaya? I asked him with a shocking face.Being Muslim he was selling Puja materials outside the Hindu temple which was something very new and strange to me.He might have read my confused face so he said haa Madamji, mere dadaji aur ram chacha bahut acche dost the.Ram chacha mandir ki safai karte the aur mere dadu yahi pe phool bechate the he told me his history.Ohh...so you are Rahim chacha's grandson? i asked him.Yes he nodded his head! So he was our Gully boy staying in the next lane.

Ram uncle and Rahim uncle's friendship was well known to the entire town.Both were thick friends,always together.Both their houses were next to each other and both the families were always available for each other in every good and bad times.Rahim uncle used to be present at every Ramleela playing the role of Laxman and Ram uncle used to help them prepare gallons of sheerkurma during Ramzan times.Entire town had immense respect for this duo.And no doubt they have imbibed the same diligence and Mutual respect for all the religions in Ibrahim too.

He got better and was discharged after a few days.Every Monday he used to go to Shivalaya very early in the morning.Clean,neatly dressed in his white kurta and payjama and netted cap on his head was his trademark dress style.He used to sweep the entire courtyard of the temple,sprinkle water and spread his washed sheets on the ground to arrange the heaps of bright,fresh colourful flowers which he used to get from General Bazaar.Different colours, different fragrances of fresh flowers used to make the temple premises more pure and divine.There were roses..pink, red, orange and the yellow roses, marigold, aboli, mogara, nishiganda and bilvapatri also.

From then on i started going to Shivalaya every Monday to pray to the Lord but more so over to check on Ibrahim's health status.After darshan i used to sit for a while under the huge banyan tree talking to Ibrahim.Dont you go to school? I asked him one day.Jaata hun na madam but Monday yaha ka kaam khatam karke 12 baje jaata hun school he told me."Mere Dadu bolte the madam, Ram kya Allah kya, jejus kya, sab insaan ko neki hi sikhate hai.Koi bhi majhab aapas mei bair karna nahi sikhata.Yeh toh log apne fayde k liye Geeta, kuran mei likhi batoon ko apne hisab se badlte hai.Khuda toh sabko ek saath khush hi dekhna chahta hai na"he enlightened me with his words.I was in the awe of his maturity towards such sensitive topics at this young age.Days passed by and i could see him getting leaner and weak.His shine in the eyes was getting dimmer and dimmer day by day.And one fine day i did not see him selling flowers.What might have happened to him? Is he alright? Or school exams?? I thought to myself and drove back to his home.His mother, Ruksana a widower welcomed me in their small abode.He is not keeping well madam, continuous cough and fever.We bought medicines from the government hospital but it's not working she added. I examined him.He was having wheeze. I sent him medications which i had at my home and told his mother not to worry about medicines as i would be sending it regularly.I bought a nebulizer and sent it to his home.Some inhaled medications would help him breath well.After that 2 weeks i was busy with my conference and couldn't go towards temple side but medicines kept reaching him regularly without fail.Within the mountain of work Ibrahim was totally lost in the chaos of my thoughts.Conference was a huge success and we the all organizers were very much delighted.Coming out of the Conference mania took me over a week's time.

After a week i entered the ICU with great zeal and here i found him.Ibrahim lying on the bed weak and fragile breathing through NRM mask,a type of non invasive ventilation.His breathing was too shallow and pulse was low. IV fluids and Ryles tube feeding were trying to keep him alive.He was fighting for his Life."His lungs are very bad mam, he is not supporting conservative management", my resident doctor updated me his condition.I could see him struggling for each and every breath.CT chest showed complete damage of the lungs.He was having multiple complications of prolonged steroid therapy.His BP was high, sugars were shooted and he had severe gastritis.I sat near his chair. He opened his eyes slowly with great difficulty and seeing me he had a faint smile on his face.Madamji...i have got flowers for you.Today is Monday, you might not have got flowers at the temple this morning.I told my Ammi to get it here so when you come to see me i can hand it over to you.He pointed towards the medicine trolly.In the lower compartment i could see fresh colourful flowers wrapped neatly in the paper.Bholenath ko mera salam kehna...Ab seede unke pass Jake hi seva karunga and he started getting breathless.We shifted him to the ventilator section and ventilated him. I knew no amount of treatment could save him now.As the sun started setting Ibrahim's breathing started sinking.With the heavy heart we bid him final goodbye.Alas on his favourite Monday he went to meet his favourite Bholenath.Now i won't be seeing this cheerful,calm and composed guy in his white kurta and netted cap sitting within the heaps of colourful flowers every Monday.Now there was none who could see me and start wrapping the flowers excitedly.I knew without Ibrahim and his flowers my Puja to the Lord will be incomplete.

Some people bring breeze of positivity and happiness in our lives.He was far above the Hindu Muslim chaos.He was true devotee who chose humanity and mankind above all.He showed us these religious tags we have labelled for ourselves but from within we all are one and the same.True feelings and emotions binds us together"His mother came to me weeping.Aapne bahut help Kari madam humari...nahi toh private hospital mei ilaaz karana nahi hota humse.Ek hafte se bimaar tha, hospital le aaye tabhi bahut serious tha,kuch ummeed nahi thi hame.Par woh ruka tha aapke liye".He wanted to meet me for the last time before he left this world."Usne mujhe bola hai mai rahu ya na rahu mere phool madam ji ke pass jarur jaane chahiye hamesha".And his mother has promised him the same.

Tears started rolling on my cheeks heavily wetting the flowers wrapped in the paper which i was holding in my hands.True...some people leaves lasting imprints on our mind and heart...like this one..!!!

* * *

CHAPTER 29
THE PATH-FINDERS

I finished my afternoon ICU rounds and went to my OPD room.Parents were waiting in the lobby for me with their kids and as i reached near my room 4-5 people suddenly got up and wished me "Salaam madam".I was jerked a bit and turned around,the family has got their kid for my consultation.Grandfather was bowing, mother was smiling at me and 2-3 kids were busy playing among themselves. I smiled at them and entered my room.They came inside, Aadab madam the baritone voice of the grandfather in his late 80's banged my ears.kaise ho aap? I asked him.With yours and God's grace I'm all fine madam.After surgery I'm doing good and he showed 3 laproscopy port marks on his abdomen beneath his kurta.He had undergone cholecystectomy a few months back.Please pray for my father in law madam, his daughter in law had requested me in their last visit.

Imam ko laaye hai dikhane said the mother.She was a young,dynamic and a very confident lady in her late 20's already with 3 kids,imam being the youngest.He was born with low immunity and was falling sick often.They have roamed across the whole city meeting many doctors but there were no signs of improvement in this child. They were very poor and weren't affording much tests and big hospital fees.When they got him for the first time to me he was barely 9 months old, very thin, malnourished,marasmic child looking very dull and not gaining weight.He gets frequent loose motions madam.. in past 2 months we have admitted him thrice.She put the records and summaries of past 3 admissions from the largest government setup in our area on my table.Repeated infections had weakened his digestive system and he was pumped with many many medications.

Why is he soo weak and fragile?he hasn't gained much weight also i said worriedly.He doesn't eat anything madam.. just like every mother's complaint she tried explaining me. I examined him thoroughly, he hasn't recieved a single vaccine shot from birth till date,not even BCG.He was all time ill madam so couldn't vaccinate she told bit sadly.He was lying still in his mother's lap not moving much.His milestones were also bit delayed due to malnutrition.First we need to control his infections, have to improve his nutrition and boost his immune power by vaccinating him so that he won't be prone for further infections i explained them in detail.They were happy that i gave them much time and answered their every small and single query.

I started working on that child. Prescribed some tests, started him on good medications,prepared a very affordable and manageable diet chart to improve his nutrition and also started early stimulation for him.Slowly and steadily he started growing and gaining weight. vaccination schedule was followed.Loose motions,cold,cough episodes were less now. Admissions were not noted.He looked alert in his next few visits and started walking with support.This developed immense faith of the family in me.It takes lots of patience and perseverance along with hardwork for a doctor to treat every patient as each case is different and challenging.

I was treating the child on one side and noting the unique relationship of daughter in law with her old father in law.Mother and her 3 children were always accompanied by her old father in law.It was more of father- daughter relationship than in laws.He was very caring about his grand children. Daughter in law was very fierce and confident lady who spoke fluent Hindi and English.She was well read but was married in a very poor house due to her circumstances.She used to call her father in law daddyji and like a very caring and doting father he used to be always supportive towards her daughter in law and grandchildren.He used to get them sweets, bun-pav,he used to play with them and he got his surgery done in a government hospital so that his grandson gets good treatment."Ab humare bache hi kitne din hai madam, Kiku itni purani outdated machine pe kharcha karna?" he used to say helplessly.In today's materialistic world where most of the daughters/ sons don't share any good relationship with their in laws, this bond looked very unique to me.

My father in law is very supportive of me madam, my husband doesn't earn much.At this age my father in law goes for work and earns to run our family.He pays my children's school fees,takes care of our entire family a lot.I lost my father in young age but i got this father instead she told with moist eyes.Respect, gratitude was flowing in her words.Truly blessed are those who gets such inlaws i felt."Madam ji se sab acche se samaz lo, medicine ka,khane ka he entered the room with vaccines while instructing his daughter-in-law.Ji Daddyji she replied.They left my cabin after imam's checkup.Few minutes later she entered briskly into my room again, madam ek request karni hai aapse.What? i asked surprisingly.Next week Daddyji ki surgery hai gall bladder ki, unke liye pray kariye, aapki dua bahut jaldi kabool hoti hai" she said with a hope. Definitely why not i told her affirmatively with a smile.

And then today they have turned up after many months for imam's vaccination again.He is grown up now 2 years old, walking on his own. Grandfather and imam's mother both entered my cabin.Thoda paise jama karne time hua iss time so ek week late hua madam he said with a grin.No problem aaj de denge vaccine i assured him.Dekho madam jab aapke pass laye the he wasn't even moving and see him today he is all running and playing around.We can't thank you much his voice trembled!

I saw imam jumping happily in his own world with his two siblings.Madam i have joined LLB,i have finished my BA before marriage and because of financial constraints and family responsibilities couldn't persue further education.But after looking and meeting you my father in law got inspired a lot.He always told me "tumhe madam jaise banna hai," you learn well and help the needy. He arranged my fee money from his PF and enrolled me in a law school she told proudly with tears rolling down her cheeks. He had got his surgery done in the government hospital and saved that amount for his daughter in law's education.You are really great i told him as he entered my room with a sweet Box. Mai toh bas apna dharam nibha raha hun madam..Beta toh padh na saka, ab beti ko pada raha hun he told proudly.I bowed him through my heart as getting to meet such genuine people nowadays is a rarity.

These people were true pathfinders.They fought with every tough situation with great courage. No complaints, no cribbing,no blaming fate.They never played a victim card for being poor,they never requested for free treatment.In every tough phase they accepted the reality,worked hard,kept patience and followed my advice.Their faith and patience gave more energy to my hardwork.In today's era there are very few people who truly appreciate others skills and hardwork and these were one among them.They found their own path and build their own destiny.They were perfect example of saying "God help those who help themselves".Chalte hai madam,bas duaaon mei yaad rakhna they said."Ab next time Advocate Amayra fatima se hi milungi mei" i told them looking at the dynamic daughter in law. Ji haan jarur ! And she left smilingly..!

* * *

CHAPTER 30

A DIALOGUE IN THE DARK

Diwali was nearing and we all were very enthusiastic about Diwali shopping.Home was cleaned,newly painted, decorations done.Dresses with matching jewellery were bought,colourful Rangolis and designs to be put in front of the door was selected.Now only shopping left was that of diyas and candles.My sister herself being an eye specialist suggested that we should buy these items from the Blind school society in her hospital campus.They do wonderful job she said.Ohh is that so..we will buy from there this time i said and our next day visit to the blind school was finalised.

The next morning we reached Blind school.It was on the same campus as the hospital where my sister was working.The campus was huge and spacy with many big trees standing tall and spreading their green branches making the sight more green.It was 9 am and melodious songs were sung in the building.As we entered we could see the blind students standing in a line and singing prayers.Their voice was melodious and prayers sounded divine "Hich aamuchi prathana Ani hech amuche magane, manasane manasashi manasa Sama vagane"they were singing.What a meaningful prayer,they were praying for entire humanity,humans should be kind and humanly towards other humans was the meaning.I was really touched!!

After prayers the principal came and greeted us,she knew my sister well.She took us to her office and offered us hot piping tea and biscuits.With fresh mind and fresh heart we walked along with the staff to meet the blind children in their workshop.This was a huge hall, children were sitting in the groups and doing their work with great zeal and pomp.They looked so happy.Although they didn't had sight they were trained so well in making candles. I was amazed to see their hands moving swiftly making candles of various shapes,sizes and fragrances.They were making scented candles,how they can make it without seeing? i asked their trainer in a jippy.We have vocational courses for them mam, they are trained in these skills so they can earn,learn and be independent. Although they can't see they can do all their works on their own right from cooking, cleaning and all other works she added.We bought as many candles as we could for our home and to gift all other relatives and friends.There was other section where they were selling scented soaps, soaps of many colours and shapes.There were fishes, elephants, birds, custard apple and many more shapes of soaps and also they had colourful rangolis,oils and scented scrub(called as uttana in Marathi and Ubtan in Hindi).Their skill of making these things were really wonderful.We bought many soaps, oils and scrubs.Our Diwali was much bright and radiant now.

On the day of Diwali Padwa we invited these blind kids to our home.We had arranged their Musical programme for our friends,relatives and dear ones.They came with Harmonium, guitar, tabla and flute.They started with Bhoopali, RamRaksha,Hanuman chalisa,bhajans and they slowly turned to classical, bollywood and even pop.It was truly amazing evening.Their show stealer was fusion of classical and

Bollywood music who ruled everyones heart.No one have ever heard such tunes.How God has gifted these kids with this amazing talent i thought.Music needs no sight or language it needs just heart to feel.We served them delicious meal,packed snack items and Diwali gifts for them.They were so happy..!! Their happiness brought joys to many lives.

We kept meeting these all kids often. Sometimes for their painting exhibition or their pottery making classes.They were technologically very advanced and have built their own road maps and navigation system in their Brail language.They invited us for their annual function as chief guest and we graced the occasion and felt honoured to appreciate these multi-talented children.Words were short to describe their skills and qualities.God forgot to give gift of sight to them but he loaded them with other versatile talents which none others with vision had.They were real visionary beyond sight.At their school gathering they did Wheelchair Dandiya, their coordination ,Swift movements of wheel chairs while playing dandiyas was too superb and beyond imagination.From where they get soo much power and strength i was puzzled.I always used to say to my sister if only they could see this world! "They see through their hearts and minds.This outer darkness is for us as they are lit from within"she told me.

To prove this true she took me to a very unique and innovative restaurant named Dialogue in the dark.We were greeted by the manager and at the entrance we were blindfolded with cloth on our eyes so we were technically blind now. We were taken to our tables and as we seated our blind Stuart came and took our order and very meticulously all the blind workers there served our dinner.They were so organised and hosted us timely.The food was tasty but more miraculous was this expirence where we could feel how their world looked without light and this memory was etched in my mind forever.

Tomorrow you have to come to my hospital in the morning with me my sister told me.We have some special function at hospital she added and kept my curiosity high.I reached there the next morning only to find it was an Eye donation campaign on the occasion of World's Sight day.We pledged to donate our eyes and then the good news broke.They have got few donated eyes which could be transplanted in these blind kids.The day came and panel of highly skilled doctors including my sister operated on them.7 children who were visually eligible were selected for this surgery.They were sitting on the chairs next to each other.Nurses came and opened their bandage on the eyes one by one.Slowly they opened their eyes.They had slight photophobia initially as the sunrays banged their cornea and then their retina.First they could see blur and then clarity of vision improve. They could see the green trees,the blue sky,rising sun,the birds whose chirping sounds they could hear daily....today they were seeing them in real.Tears rolled down their cheeks.Our nurse incharge patted their back emotionally,Mary sister they screamed with happiness.You are Mary sister na they asked with joy.They could recognise everyone with their touch,they hugged us and expressed their gratitude.

They felt we were more,more,more beautiful when they saw us alas it was conection by our hearts,direct Dil se.And this was the turning point for my sister which motivated her to work relentlessly for these blinds and needy,motivating the people to take care of their eyes and to encourage them to donate their eyes so that others can see this beautiful world through our eyes and we can remain immortal forever.And what can be more pure,more joyous and more noble than this !!

* * *

CHAPTER 31
LITTLE MISS SUNSHINE

I walked out of "Moms and Me" carrying the huge box of gift wrapped in a shiny wrapper and drove happily to the "PLAZA", the biggest and Posh convention centre of my town.As i reached the venue the turban clad person in black safari came forward to assist me " it's vallet parking,keys please" he said smilingly. I got down off my car and my eyes were taken aback with the beautiful decor and huge lightings brightening the garden hall.The huge chandeliers were hanging sprinkling their cool beams making atmosphere more cooler. Colourful flowers were hanging and stage was decorated with balloons, glitters and cartoon cutpieces making it more grand. It was indeed a royal affair!! A huge 3 layered cake was put in between and name on it read as "Happy birthday Little Miss Sunshine "!!The name brought big smile on my face as i have given this name to this tiny tot, her parents looked beamingly happy.Miss Sunshine looked very pretty and elegant in her wings wala pari dress.Happy birthday song was played and the hall was echoed with claps and Laughters.Dance,games, thambola arranged brought fun and frolic to one and all.After a year long of sorrows, worry, grief and tensions, this day had brought joys and happiness into their dark world.I greeted them all, handed over the gift and went to the lavish dinner spread. Each and every arrangement there showed their ecstacy after passing the gloomy days.She turned ONE today! A born fighter she is i said to myself and this very thought took me down my memory lane where i first saw her in the critical phase of life and death.

Madam I'm getting one very sick baby...keep ventilator ready our registrar from satellite centre called me in panicky. His voice was soo muffled in harsh ambulance siren,the sound of red light on the ambulance always makes us hyperalert and till the case reached us we were ready with warm warmer, B- CPAP blender, a ventilator, crash trolley and what not.Fully drenched in sweat our registrar carried the tiny baby in his hands and very thin stick like sister bagging the ET tube came panting along with him as if she required ambu bag breaths more than the baby itself. Escorted them was the ambulance driver who lifted the oxygen cylinder and walked behind them and he was the one who waited patiently till initial stabilisation is done as he never budge unless we return him his oxygen prongs.

Our Registrar doctor kept the baby in the warmer and spoke heavily..i went at the last moment madam, unbooked case it was, baby did not cry at birth, intubated with great difficulty and immediately shifted here he updated me and before i respond anything he fleeted the scene dumping all the responsibility on my shoulder.Baby was sick and her breathing was heavy we started her on ventilator, IV Fluids,antibiotics and other supportive treatment. I called father and counselled him regarding the condition of his baby. Young father was confused as he was very naive to this kind of situation and said whatever possible you do but save my baby. When i was examining the baby we were shocked to see that there is no anal opening to this girl,her clitoris was very large and her genitals looked ambiguous (difficult to identify if it's male or female genitals). Again we counselled the parents for this condition,now listening to these all complaints poor father got more scared and worried. He started sweating and trembling,tears started rolling down his cheeks.We had a very hard time getting this baby mam, baby's mother had 4 abortions. They said it's related to APLA syndrome, she conceived after 3 failed IUI, she had high BP and on the verge of throwing fits.Her sugars shot up from second trimester we had been through a lot till we come here please do something but save my baby he was pleading. I could sense his anxiety being father for the first time and getting to know so many problems on day 1 itself is really very very traumatic.

We sent the special hormonal tests and did the sonography for internal organs and were glad there was uterus and ovaries correlating with outer female genitals. We told the father the baby is girl only and confirming the sex of child father felt bit relieved. But his journey was too far, baby had no anal opening and had to undergo surgery for the same. Days on ventilator,IVF and TPN, antibiotics and ionotropes the treatment was done but course was long. Slowly as time moved baby was getting stabilised on ventilator and we could come down on pressure and oxygen requirment but suddenly on day 5 of her life baby started desaturating,oxygen level decreased rapidly and heart rate slowed down. Within seconds the baby was pale and shocky!

My experienced mind told me it was another life threatening complication i brought the torch and did the transillumination test bedside.Yes there was an air leak. Xray chest also confirmed the same diagnosis. The baby's right chest had massive pneumothorax (air in the chest cavity) immediately the needle was put in the second intercostal space and the air was drained a bit.Emergency intercostal chest tube was placed and air was drained. Slowly heart rate increased, colour improved and limp listless baby started moving.Sometimes these small babies will have spontaneous air leaks leading to life threatening condition.This baby was blessed to survive all such major blows.

Gradually baby improved with time. Now baby was extubated to oxygen and then to room air.Slowly Ryles tube feeding was started and later baby started accepting spoon feeds well.Her journey from 1.3 kgs to 1.8 kgs was truly adventurous with lots of ups and downs still she survived this tsunami. She was a real fighter !! The baby was off oxygen and off the monitoring system and ready for discharge. For the first time the father held his baby in his hand, the warm soft touch of his baby bloomed his face.He thanked us a ton for saving the life of his precious baby.We wrapped the baby in a warm blanket, they took her in arms and started walking.The baby looked calm and soo peaceful that peace radiated to us as well.The satisfaction of saving a critical baby and sending them home Hale and hearty is happiness of different level which cannot be measured but only treasured and that's the beauty of my profession!! And thats why I named this baby Little Miss Sunshine who tide all her life's odd like a true fighter and brought light,hope and happiness in her parents lives !!

* * *

CHAPTER 32

LOVE YOU ZINDAGI

Life is like a kaleidoscope of infinite expirences.Some moments of joys,some sorrows, thrill, excitement, pain, agonies and what not. As a doctor in this Journey called Life we meet innumerable patients and with each new patient and every new expirence some part of us is grown again.And this one story is worth penning down as it is a story of courage, faith, perseverance and determination which proved that a strong will power and determination can literally move the mountains!

This was like any other morning hours of my hustly bustly life.Alarm buzzing at six, jumping out of my bed, enjoying cool breeze in my balcony with hot cuppa of tea in my hands, brief walk and glance through the newspaper, instructing maid and cook for their daily chores and then getting ready for my hospital in the speedy way to reach the NICU bang on time. Really Doctor's life is not an easy task at all.Its like walking on a tight rope balancing personal and professional life and moreover balancing your physical and mental sanctity too! As I was hurriedly getting ready for my hospital duty my phone rang.Mam,one 5 days baby got admitted now, baby is unresponsive and limp.I immediately rushed to the hospital only to find a very sick baby in comatose state, breathing faintly.We ventilated the baby immediately started ivf, antibiotics and Bp maintaining medicines. Plan of treatment and investigations were instantly chalked out.

What happened to the baby, why the baby is like this? from when? I asked parents concerndly.Weeping father said Don't know madam, baby was normal till day 3 of life. From yesterday baby was constantly sleeping, dull, not accepting feeds.Pediatrician there did the blood test which was normal but since this morning baby is not responding at all so rushed here.

History noted,Investigation reports traced. Infection markers were negative, electrolytes,calcium, magnesium was normal, Liver function test showed mild elevation of enzymes.CT scan brain just showed cerebral edema,no evidence of any bleed. My brain started connecting the dots.Inborn error of metabolism was thought and plasma ammonia,lactate and few higher investigations like TMS and Gcms were sent. And to our dismay ammonia was highly elevated and was in1000's. In no time we got to know we were dealing with a very rare and complex disease of Urea cycle defect where Liver fails to handle ammonia produced in our body.TMS and Gcms report supported our diagnosis.Genetic study was done which confirmed, it was Citrullinemia type 1.

Reports devastated the entire family and even us because it was the rarest form of the disease with no medical cure. Only chance of survival was with Liver transplantation with a very guarded prognosis. This treatment was obviously out of reach for many people in India who struggle hard to meet their ends.

With great disappointment we counselled the parents about the disease and told that there is no treatment other than Liver Transplantation and doing such a major and difficult surgery that too in such a small baby was highly tedious and literally near to impossible.

But still the parents were determined and were ready to go till any extent for treating their child. "Go ahead Mam, do what so ever is possible for our baby, result is in HIS hands but we want to try till very end, parents spoke affirmatively.

The baby started with a Metabolic cocktail, a special therapy for such kids.Sodium Benzoate and Arginine was procured making our pharmasist to run from one centre to another. Finally we were shining in our armours getting ready for a difficult battle of saving this baby from a very rare and difficult disease. In this disease we have to completely restrict the proteins and it's very difficult for the baby to survive without proteins as they are the building blocks of our body cells.

Slowly baby improved on the ventilator, started moving and opening the eyes and was weaned off from the ventilator.Now the biggest challenge was feeding this baby as his liver was not going to tolerate dietary proteins and any protein would lead to high ammonia levels again.Dietician opinion was taken and baby was started on special diet with very minimal proteins.But to our despair baby's ammonia instantly shooted to 2000 and above and baby crashed again and went into coma. Again we were back to square one.We told the parents regarding poor prognosis and bleak outcome. But they were rock steady in their decision and wanted us to do our very best.

Now this case was a real challenge to us.We continued with sodium benzoate, arginine and consulted nutritonist for zero protein diet.The special diets were specially ordered from Banglore.And this fighter baby still continued to fight for his survival.With parents determination to continue the treatment, our hard work and unending efforts baby slowly started tolerating special formula feeds.As the baby stabilized slowly very small amount of proteins were introduced.Days were passing and our struggle to keep the baby alive was continued.

Many Gastroenterologist and Hepatologist were consulted from Hyderabad,Delhi and Mumbai who unanimously told Liver Transplant being the only treatment for this condition without which baby would not survive.But Liver Transplant in such a small baby of only one month...So complex..!!

Our search began to find which hospital can do Liver Transplant in such a tiny tot.

All the leading institutes of India where Liver Transplant was done were hesitant to operate in such a young boy. Everyone advised us to wait till 6-9 months of age for surgery.Now the challenge was big in front of us how to survive this baby till that age as any minor infection would decompensate baby's liver and land him on the ventilator again.

After lots of background research,a hospital in Chennai was discovered with a well known doctor doing Liver Transplant in small babies as well. His expertise was vast and results were good. But so many problems were still challenging us and saga continued. Who will donate the Liver? How to transport the baby to chennai?

Again the determinative parents took the lead.Matching donor was found.With lots of tensions, insecurities and doubts in their minds and after lots of counselling and moral support from me and our team finally they made their mind.Now main question was how to transport?Road journey was time consuming and troublesome, flight journey was risky.

We evaluated pros and cons and decided to air lift the baby.Multiple trials were given to check for his lung status if baby was suitable to fly. And then we formulated a team and succesfully Airlifted the baby from Hyderabad to Chennai !

After torrendous Medical journey and battery of tests finally baby was taken up for the Liver transplant.The fear, anxiety, stress was seen in the eyes of baby's parents.Future was uncertain but their Will power was strong! After 7-8 hours of long surgery finally the baby was transplanted with the new liver.Baby was now leased with the New life!!

Hundreds and thousands of prayers were going for the baby from me, my team, fellow colleagues, our entire nursing staff and nonetheless the baby's entire family. All were praying with just one thought that baby should tide this crisis soon.

This brave little warrior again fought the stormy icu period post surgery and slowly recovered, got weaned off from the ventilator, started accepting the feeds and then was discharged in a stable condition. That moment when the teary eyed mother cuddled her baby who touched the heaven steps and came back again in her lap was just incredible! These moments cannot be described in the words but just can be felt.No words spoken but only emotions spoke the volume. It was the highest dedication and sacrifice of the parents for their baby.Their entire family stood rock steady with them in this journey. Really parents love cannot be measured but can only be treasured.

This baby is a real fighter,fighting his life's all odd. His parents are really great showing so much patience and perseverance who never gave up on their child despite so much negative counselling and poor prognosis explained.With all the extreme efforts and hard work taken by me and my team and the surgical team in this case today I feel so glad and so proud to see the baby surviving with such a grace and Elan.These moments really impart million dollar satisfaction and there is no other joy seeing your hardwork paying off soo well!

Yes it's rightly said God helps those who help themselves. And this baby increased my faith many folds in the concept "Yes with unconditional, persistent efforts with positive mindset Miracles do happen.Definitely like this one!!!

. . .

This baby is indeed a Medical miracle to survive such a tough battle and I'm glad I could impart my knowledge,skills, experience and clinical acumen to make this baby smile back again.That's why I felt this baby loves his life very much and so Life loves him back manifolds.So friends we have to love our life because we have got only one to live here.No doubt this journey was terrifically Memorable!!!

* * *

CHAPTER 33

DIL DHADAKNE DOO

It's so miraculous & joyous to see the heart rate of the baby in Nicu reverting back to normal after a bad SVT. A term baby weighing 2.7kgs was delivered via Lscs & was admitted for the breathing difficulty. Initial investigations revealed positive infection markers and hence the baby was started on antibiotics after sending the blood culture.Baby started improving with the treatment but required oxygen support albiet a little longer.Gradually baby recovered,got on to the full feeds.Mother was involved in the baby care and we were planning for the baby's discharge next day. The very next day in my morning round I found out baby's heart rate to be very high (280 beats/min) although baby was active. Bedside diagnosis of Supraventricular tachycardia was done.

Baby was observed for sometime and as heart rate continued to be high ECG was taken which confirmed our diagnosis.Baby was then treated with injection Adenosine.I was hoping to see the miracle as its known that majority of SVT's revert within a single shot of adenosine. The full team was ready with an enthusiastic nursing brother to assist me in the rapid push of the drug and NS by 3 way technique.One shot over and we waited for normalcy of the heartrate. But no it didn't happen so again the full team was enthusiastically ready for the second attempt and we all were hoping atleast this go will be fruitful. Adenosine rushed and we eagerly waited to see if heartrate comes back to normal.Time lapsed but heartrate didn't normalise.Heart rate of my nursing staff started sinking as they started loosing hopes.I told them not to loose hope but just pray and went ahead with third and last dose of adenosine.But chances to see the rare medical miracle of heart rate normalising after adenosine was just getting bleaker. I waited patiently just praying the thought to turn out to be true.Time was running and i couldn't see heart rate decresing anytime sooner. My mind started mental mapping for the other drugs to settle the heart rate by now.Books said adenosine causes miraculous reversal of SVT almost instantaneously but in our case luck was not on our side. More the rapid heart rate was for a very long time, chances of cardiac failure and sudden cardiac arrest were high. Just like it's said "Der aaye Durust aaye"heart rate started dropping slowly..280...270...254.....213......204.......188......176...168....154..

As heart rate started dropping the adrenaline rush got infused in our nursing staff and they screamed with joy "Mam heart rate normalised! I was overjoyed too to see this miraculous conversion of tachycardia to normalcy. We took the cardiologist's opinion and the baby was continued with oral drugs to keep the heart rate under check. Baby was observed for couple of days and then was dicharged in stable condition.Although Neonatal SVT's are rare,one should have keen observation and timely intervention to avoid the future havock. Although it's said SVT's revert rapidly with adenosine sometimes it may take longer.The tension and anxiety on the parents face as we told them regarding SVT and then the lines of smile created as we announced regarding the reversal of tachycardia were unforgetful. Being Doctors and especially working in the critical areas of ICU's the moments of utmost happiness is nothing but to save a life. Just two words from the overjoyed teary eyed parents..i.e.." Thanks Doctor" makes you forget all the stress and tiredness you bored for them all the way.And i think that's the beauty of being a doctor.

* * *

CHAPTER 34

THE RAINBOW OF LIFE

I drove from the countryside and reached my colony. It's mid june past yet no traces of rains.Mansoon was delayed this year. As i reached my colony road it became dark and cold. The sky was full with clouds and wind made dry leaves to fly in the air. Rain would start anytime now. I hurriedly parked my car in my parking slot and as i entered my house it started pouring heavily. I made hot tea and started making onion pakodas. It's the best tea time recipe in the rainy season and no Maharashtrian would ever miss this chance of eating piping hot pakoda along with hot ginger tea during the beautiful rainy evening.

After awaiting soo long this was the first heavy rains of this Mansoon. I turned my radio on.Soft melodious rain songs in the background, hot piping tea and tasty mouthwatering onion fritters and continuous rains outside...Ahha what a combination to treasure! I came and sat in my soft chair next to my favourite french window. After soo many days I was feeling so relaxed and free.Feeling of liberation is what i was expirencing now in the right sense.

Some sound near my front door broke my thought process.

There was some movement near the door. I went to the front door and saw from the window pane. A poor lady was trying to protect herself from the pouring rain. She was totally drenched and was holding her small baby tightly to her chest covering with her saree pallu.I told my maid to take her bit inside so she can be saved from the heavy downpour. She sat in one corner looking scared and worried for her little baby. She had some thick cement bag in her hand. I made her to sit on the mat and told my maid to give her old towel to dab herself and her baby dry. I pulled out some old saree from the wardrobe and told her to change. I was more worried about her little one. I told my maid to bring some hot tea and bhajji for her. By now she was bit warm and her shivering has come down.I went inside and brought some warm milk to her baby. Her eyes were filled with tears. Madam I don't have enough words to thank you.No one even let us to stand near their door but you not only gave us shelter in this heavy rains but also offered us to eat and she started crying.

Don't feel bad. Its really spine chilling cold outside.I can't see a small baby suffering in this kind of rain.Give her some milk she may be hungry. She took the milk glass from my hand and put some milk in the old vessel of hers. Slowly she took out one small puppy from the cement bag which she was carrying with her. Puppy was also fully drenched and was shivering.She offered him some warm milk and wiped him dry with her old saree. Puppy drank milk and sat close to her taking warmth from her body in the chilling cold environment.Then she fed her baby with great affection.Baby looked tierd, she drank milk and fell asleep.I was moved by this lady's gesture. From where did you got this puppy? I asked curiously. His mother was accompanying us everywhere madam. She protected us all the time. We shared our little food what we got daily. She died recently and left this puppy behind. Now it's our turn to care for her little one she told me with tears rolling on her cheeks. My heart cried out to see such a humanitarian nature of this poor lady who didn't knew if she could feed herself daily but was taking care of these two babies together. Really this lady was poor by money but rich by heart.

So from where you are? Where is your family? I enquired. Madam parents are no more. Grandmother raised me and married me off at a very young age. Husband was not a good man and I suffered a lot with him. When i got this baby she was born blind so my husband abandoned me and my child.And then on I'm roaming this village to that staying in temples and eating what I get...she told her story. I have studied till 9th standard madam, I want to work and earn.I dont want to be dependant on anyone she told sobbing.

Let me see the baby once i asked her. I took the torch and threw torch light in her eyes. There was this white opaque dot in the eyes making the child unable to see. A father can abandon his child but the mother cannot do this to her baby at any cost.Good,bad or disabled mother loves her child equally. I checked her eyes thoroughly and was sure it was congenital cataract. I told her it can be cured with surgery and should try for it. She was shocked and glad to know that there is some bleak chance that her baby can see this beautiful world.

I called my sister who is renowed ophthalmologist and told her the whole story. She suggested me that we can take her to the Government hospital where the baby can be treated free of cost. I made her arrangement in a nearby Ashram hostel where she was assured of safe stay and good food. I regularly visit this place every month for health checkups and knew these management people well. Next day my sister came and examined the baby and confirmed it was congenital cataract.We took the baby to the Anterior segment department and evaluated the baby in detail. It was an operable case and we did all the required formalities.My sister made sure that the best lenses were ordered for this baby.Date of surgery was allotted. Mother, baby and puppy were staying in Aashram and the mother started working with some clerical job in Ashram itself. Puppy also started gaining weight as he was fed regularly and taken care of. Whenever we used to visit Aashram puppy used to jump with joy and wag his tail to welcome us. He never used to leave me and used to accompany me wherever I go the whole day.

Today was the day of the surgery and mother looked very scared.The very thought of the surgery on her small child was indeed a big thing for her. But she had lot of trust on us and was sure we will do our best for her baby. Surgery was successful and new intraocular lenses were inserted in her eyes. After 2-3 days the bandage was opened and child smiled looking at her mother's face. Mother's face beamed with happiness and joy. Tears of joys started rolling on her cheeks. It was the golden moment to capture.That day the women cried her heart out. It was a new day and new life for both of them. Little puppy was also dancing with joy wagging her tail around them. Unknowingly our eyes also started flowing.This was a rare moment of content, joy and happiness. After a while mother brought the kid to us and said mam you have given her new lease of life. I cant repay your debt in this life atleast. You both are god sent to us. We named the child Roshni which means light. This child has brought the new light of hope and happiness to her mother. Their dark world started shining bright.

From then the mother regularly visit my home every sunday and helps me in gardening my plants. It's the little act of gratitude towards me she says.All the bills can't be paid in the form of money but some bills are to be paid with emotions. Compassion and kindness are the only things which can make this world really a better place to stay. In this world of pretenance and cruelty its hard to trust anyone but sometimes weighing the pros and cons of the situation and helping others in the right way can save someone's life. Little act of kindness can change someone's life forever. Today was sunday and sharada was watering my plants,her child was playing on the green grass carpet in the garden and little puppy was dancing freely everywhere.All the happy faces were around filling the happiness and peace in the air. With her new eyes little roshni was seeing the new world and the rainbow of her life. I took my camera and captured this beautiful kodak moment to cherish forever!

* * *

CHAPTER 35

JEENA ISI KA NAAM HAI

It's 7.30 am.Monday blues...Alaram buzzing continuously reminding me to get up from the bed.Door bell started ringing.Cook time! I got up with the heavy eyes,opened the door and went to freshen up.On my return back i was delighted to see a hot cup of coffee on my table.The hottness of coffee and it's aroma aurosed my sleeping senses and made my heavy head very light.One has to be very lucky to get hot coffe or tea readymade in your hands early in the morning. I thanked my cook for the piping hot coffee.You work so hard madam you too need some rest,she said with a smile! I was glad atleast some one noticed my hard work and busy life.

Next door bell rang indicating my second maid's entry.She started brooming hurriedly as it was almost 8.15am by now.I said Wow you came whooping 15 mins early Radha that's really great.I should really pat your back for this i said chukingly.She started laughing."What mam you too"..she was amused to see my changed reaction onto the lighter note today instead of daily scoldings to her for being late everyday. She broomed and mopped the floors very well and made utensils crystal clear that day!

I whroomed in the parking lot of my hospital, reached Nicu and did my rounds.Till i finish i got a call.Madam early morning one teenage girl has got admitted with seizures, please have a look.Our Emergency room doctor informed. I went upstairs in the room to meet her.I could see a teenage girl lying pale on the bed. Visible stress flowing on her face and she was having continuous twitching on her face and the body.I hold her hands.It was icy cold.So how are you feeling now? i asked her concernedly. Don't worry you will be fine. But tell me what's happening to you. My warm handshake relieved her anxiety a bit.Her eyes were teary.Mam I'm having these twitchings continuously she showed her face retracting while she spoke pointing with her hand.She was conscious and well oriented. In the night she was given Anticonvulsants and advised MRI brain. I knew by now it was not seizures.As all that glitters is not gold likewise all the symptoms seen cannot be pathological.Many of them are psychological too! It's more of psychosomatic diseases on rise now. And I have to dig into her history with her mother to find out the cause.You are all fine i said.When are your exams ? It was there yesterday but I missed my final exam mam.I'm doing final year B-pharmacy she said softly. Ok..no issues. You be alright first.Don't worry about your exams now. You will be fine very soon I said to her assuringly.She looked bit relieved!

I went out of the room and met the mother who was waiting near the nursing station.How is my daughter madam? She never had this kind of episode any time earlier.She will be alright na? She asked crying.Don't stress her much and she will be okay. It's all stress related i told the mother. Nothing other than that na madam I'm very worried about her exams.She missed it.She looked very worried.I said no issues she can write exams later but you will not get another chance to build a good rapport with your daughter again after this i told her. Why she is soo stressed? Any triggering factors? I was now inquisitive to know the cause behind this condition of hers.

Madam we are 6 sisters, Mother started her story. Our father left us as we all daughters were born to him. My mother was tierd of his daily blamegames. He went one fine day and never returned. My mother from being a very conservative Muslim family raised us alone. She had struggled a lot for us, worked very hard. She did job in those times madam when Muslim Women were not allowed to even step out of our houses.She educated all of us.I'm tutor and take home tutions. My elder sister is Economy professor and all other sisters are also well educated and well placed. I too have three daughters only madam and my husband also left me and eloped with some one else. Now I'm worried about my daughters.How their life will be? I don't want them to suffer and hence I keep poking them to study well. I feel so happy when my students fair well in the exams. And when i see my daughters not studying well i keep scolding them. I feel what will they do if they don't study well and won't be independent and she started crying.

Now i understood the whole scenario. Mother had insecure childhood and had struggled to study hard and survived on her own. And now seeing her daughters in her place was making her more insecure and so she was forcing them to study hard and excel.This was making her daughter stressed out and mentally drained trying to live upto her mother's expectations. And this entire thing was taking a toll on her mental status leading to psychological issues.I counselled mother not to put undue pressure on her children.After all they should be happy in their lives.Let them learn and be what they want to. Many small courses will fetch you decent money nowdays.They should love their profession and enjoy their work.Atlast their happiness is of utmost important.Your undue worry will make them more stressful.Be positive and happy in front of your kids, develop easy friendly bond with them and they will bloom i told her. She also was convinced by now.I took her slowly in her daughter's room, moved the curtain and showed her. Her girl was looking out from the window, a squirrel was dancing on the front tree. Her twitchings have disappeared and their was faint smile on her face. Stress is causing her psychological issues.You be stress free and make her stress free and she will be absolutely fine.Mother nodded her head with a sigh of relief seeing her daughter calm and composed.

We came out the room and then i saw a very old lady in 90's walking slowly with a walker. She was fragile and pale. Her silver hair spoke about her huge experience with life. A young short fair nurse was walking beside her holding her arms.I smiled at her and asked how are you granny? You feeling ok.? She smiled brightly and said yeah much better now. Her smile was too infectious. I appreciated her by saying your smile is very beautiful granny keep smiling always and all your illness will run away. It brightened her face and she started walking with full energy. My few words increased few grams of flesh on her body.

The mother of that teenage girl was watching this from behind. She came after me and said madam will you come and meet my daughter daily? Your words are very encouraging and lively. It's adding hope and cheerfulness to everyone's life. I smiled with a big yes.i went daily to the wards for the next few days to spend time with the teenage girl and granny. Both recovered really fast. Along with medicine these small words of love and care creates miracles and wonders in others lives. Most of the people are more devoid of love than anything else.They just need someone to hear them out and care for them.

On the day of the discharge girl ringed herself on our Nicu landline from her ward and invited me for a cup of tea. The old granny from the next room joined us too.The room which was dark,bleak and sorrowful a few days ago was lit up in the laughter now. I could see two generations poles apart sitting beside me on my both sides.One side was the young child trying to find out good days for her life and other side was old granny trying to find few good moments to add to her remaining days. I could see smiles on the two extremes of life. I felt as light as cottony clouds. No wonder tea tasted extra sweet that day and i was happy that i could be the light in someone else's life! So Keep smiling and spreading happiness as world needs it more. Few words of compassion and care is all that is needed to make a world happier place to live!!

* * *

CHAPTER 36
THE BORDERLESS WORLD

"We would like to have you as a chief guest for our Women's day programme", Dr Hanumanth Rao sir a well known Developmental Pediatrician who has been recently conferred with prestigious Padmashri Award from the Government of India was speaking from the other side on phone.It was indeed my honour to get invited for such an important event.Cheif guest for International Women's Day programme and that too at Sweekar Academy which was working relentlessly for the children with Mental disabilities and those with Autism,the very thought was superly nostalgic.I readily agreed!I reached the venue on time that day and walked along the campus of Sweekar Academy.It was a huge yet very very old building needing some urgent renovation and maintainence.The look of the building echoed the longetivity of the work which was going on here for ages.Huge entrance led to the small cabins of the therapists where they spoke with patients and their attenders and counselled them regarding the required treatment.On the first floor front side were the therapy rooms well equipped with various amenities for ADHD children who lacked attention and concentration.Sand

Therapy, Ball therapy, Light therapy and many more were included to increase their concentration level and memory power.The teachers were simple,humble and fully dedicated to their work and belonged from all over the India.Right from West Bengal to kerala and from Delhi, Bihar, Maharashtra to Telangana it seemed like a Mini India to me.Every teacher was soo dedicated and had passion for their work which reflected every single minute through the words they spoke.

Behind these therapy rooms were huge class rooms for students enrolled for multiple courses like bachelors and masters in intellectual disabilities, Diploma and M.Phil in Clinical psychology, Bachelor and Masters in Audiology and many more.On the ground floor behind the main building was huge Garden with a beautiful temple in the centre and a huge Auditorium for their various Cultural and Academic events. Beside the Auditorium was the school for children with the special needs. They did not only teach them theoretical things but also were giving them vocational and occupational training to make these kids self dependent.They were taught yoga, they were trained into paper and quilt art and I could see various colourful wall hangings and other artistic things made by these special kids.They were also learning simple stitch on the sewing machine.The moment i entered their classroom they greeted me Good morning maaaammm...in a loud chorus.They looked so happy to meet their new guest and they sang songs and told many interesting stories in their babbling interrupted tone.

The teachers in this school for special children were really selfless and taught them whole heartedly. It needs really a verg very big heart to accept these kind of kids who do not understand anything about the real world and were dependant on others for everything small and big. These teachers took them for physiotherapy, fed them, taught them to sing and dance and created a world of joy for them. Really making a happy world for these disable and destitutes is not a simple thing and needs lots of courage and compassion!

After strolling through the huge campus we walked to the Auditorium located centrally surrounded by some lush green garden.The stage was well decorated with hangings of all the super women from India who have excelled in their respective fields.Seeing my picture hanging amidst them was such a feel good phenomena. Inspiring and touching other life is indeed a great noble act.We were done with the Felicitation programme. By noon all the staffs too were felicitated for their dedicated work towards these special kids. It was astonishing to see more than 95 % staff working here were females.Managing their homes,kids and personal lives they were happily available here to help these kids full time.There was no frown, no frustration about handling these slow and developmentally delayed children but what they had was heart full of compassion and affection! Cultural programmes were really rocking with all the women power dancing to the beats of melodious telgu songs which instantly changed the atmosphere of the auditorium making it more vibrant and jubiliant.The Fashion show of Mentally challenged children was the show stellar and their teachers were also too active in this fashion show making them look more beautiful.One child was teacher, one was doctor,someone was mother Teresa,another one was Kalpana Chawla and many more. Here they lived many lives in one.

After sumptous lunch I walked along with one of the counsellor to her room.A child with learning disability was brought by their parents."He hates studying,he starts crying once he sees the book,his grades are constantly falling mother was complaining endlessly. Her worry about her kid was clearly seen on her face and was rationale.His IQ test was quiet disappointing.Counsellor counselled her in the best possible way and the need of special training to increase his concentration was told to them.Hearing about the fees which were undoubtedly quiet meager mother's frustration rose. If only he would have studied properly we would not have come here, she said angrily.They needed some time to decide and they left. It kept me thinking why we all Indian parents assess our children only on the marks and grades given by a particular school? Is the formal education only parameter of child's intelligence? In which ICSC school did our grandparents and parents study? Yet they are soo intelligent and have learnt many difficult life lessons from their school of expirence.They were tough enough to handle life's any crisis strongly, they never were depressed nor frustrated with their difficulties but handled them with courage and grace.Formal education is important but we should stimulate our children and encourage them to bring their best out and let them excel in their field of choice. All successful people in the world were not rank 1 student but they had passion for their work and they worked crazily hard to achieve their goals. Creative people are indeed crazy. A child can be world famous guitarist, musician, dancer, cloth weaver,designer, chef, a talented agriculturist, writer, traveller and what not...talents are borderless and no borders or boundaries can ever dim the child's inner shine. Just we need to let them glow!

It was dusk by now and it was my time to leave the campus.Programme was over and the organisers came to leave me till my car. These special kids came to wave me goodbye,they all looked soo happy and radiant.Today's all the fun activity had energised them to core.Madammmm they all said in a chorus and gave me a folded paper.I opened it just to find my beautiful picture sketched by one of them.I was totally amazed to see this extraordinary drawing skill. Same nose,same hairdo and same sparkling eyes full of life. Who says they are slow?they are brilliant and have amazing skills.I started my car and drove far. I still could see their faint images with background of setting sun waving me good bye in the side mirror. Handicapped children, children with cerebral palsy, Down's syndrome, children with hyperactivity, attention deficit,learning disabilities,Autism all were here together as a family.They did not know what their illness was but all were together here to "BE HAPPY". It was really a borderless world...no borders of caste,creed, religion,no gender discrimination, no one was more intelligent or less, no rich and no poor.It was the world of just the simple, plain adorable people.People who were just humans helping each other to be happy.It was a different world wherein all these differently abled children were caring,sharing,eating,playing together. There were no thoughts of profit or gains, no ideas to bring others down,no double standards or dirty politics.They were just innocent beautiful souls away from these dark mushy world living in peace and harmony.I thought to myself.. only if all our lives were similarly peaceful and harmonious. After all everyone wants to be happy and at peace in their lives.

It was good on the part of Indian government to recognise these kinds of work and appreciate it by bestowing prestigious award. But more than that these kids requires helping hands, hearing ears,Cheerful heart and empathetic vision to accept them as they are, just like any other normal being.Yeah it's absolutely ok to be different because varitey makes life colourful.Kudos to the people who sensed their requirement and built such an empire to support these kids and gave them their home where they feel happy and safe. I knew internally that these few people who are taking care of these special kids are God sent who are striving to create a better world for these kids to live in. My heart bowed in gratitude and utmost respect for these people with golden heart.The evening looked more divine and blissful now!

* * *

CHAPTER 37
THE VISIBLE GODS

It was a new monday morning and 9 am past. Trying to overcome monday blues i hurriedly fleeted to my nicu.The moment i entered the ICU it felt soo different.Wards were decorated,colorful balloons hanging on the walls, all nurses with smiling cheerful faces were wishing me in a chorus " Happy Doctor's day madam".I felt i have entered some Ukg or 1st std class listening to that surwala wish.Followed instantly was the yummy cake and high tea.Many messages bubbled on my mobile screen wishing Happy Doctors day and telling how doctors were second god or god like. I smiled at them and replied Thanks but we are not gods,we are the humans trained and skilled to save lives. If you see us as humans,you will treat us as humans...period!

Looking around the violence doctors are facing at work,the mistreatment and disrespect they are getting nowadays and tornado of negativity the false media is spreading these kind of wishes are losing it's charm.Yet we doctors are standing tall against all the odds and continuing our selfless service of saving lives.

Amidst all these havoc, the media and political minded people are creating against the doctors and the entire medical fraternity i must say some doctors are like Gods really! And pondering deep down the memory lane are the few names etched on my mind ever and forever remains so.

Still i remember my green days from green banglore and which tops among these are my Kidwai days.Kidwai hospital is renowned cancer hospital of banglore with huge clean arena of green trees and there i found this name with aura bigger and taller than he himself Dr Appaji and i believe there is hardly any doctor in banglore or in the entire karnataka who doesn't know him.A well known hemato-oncologist and a man with a golden heart.It's amusing to see his grand welcome in the wards daily.His little patients waiting eagerly for his visit.He is the only doctor perhaps for whom his small patient's waits eagerly throughout the morning and the moment they see him there is one adrenaline rush in these kids and the whole campus gets echoed with continuous chants of Appaji sir bandroo,Appaji sir bandroo..(appaji sir came).They run for him,hug him tight,sway to his arms,cling him and walk with him front,back,sides and everywhere shouting happily Appaji sir bandroo...Its like a welcome note and message to the other kids in the wards to take their position and sit in their bed. Daily to recieve such a warm welcome with grand procession that person should be really special! And why not his simplicity, vast knowledge and huge dedication makes him exceptional.He single handedly ran the show.Being the apex cancer institute of Karnataka there are these sea of patients.

These young kids with variety of cancers blood cancer,bone cancer,Liver cancers, metastasis in the brain,lymphomas...cruel disease wriggling young lives.And yet Dr Appaji is the ray of hope for them.I have seen him toiling selflessly the whole day. He enters the opd sharp at 9 am and keep seeing his countless patients tierdlessly beyond lunch hours. His vast clinical acumen and practical expirence won't miss a single sign. Middle of his examining patients he keep teaching us the types and the grading of cancer and the treatment related to it.In few minutes of his seeing and talking to his patients you can see his compassion flowing.We used to be hungry and tierd by noon but this young man in his late 60's keeps continuing his hundreds of OPD patients without a wrinkle on his forehead. If you enter Kidwai wards it doesn't give you the feel of the cancer ward at all.You won't find any grumpy faces there nor anyone worrying about their future. There is a world full of life,a strength to overcome their dark aliment with broad smile on their faces.You can see the tender kids accepting their cancerous life happily and radiating their happiness around.They know their number of chemotherapy cycles,they know when their lumbar puncture is due.They readily update you "Appaji sir,awunu puttaswamy radiation k hoggidane...ivathu avandu radiation day alwa...(today is the radiation day of putaswamy so he has gone for radiotherapy).Even the metastasis in the brain cannot deter their determination to live.

And Dr Appaji is pillar of strength for them.They know till Dr Appaji is for them they will live their life in full swing. He is available even in the nights for them. If some boy or girl gets serious in the night he is personally available transfusing blood,frozen plasma and monitoring that kid whole night without a blink. The moment you open the page of their casesheet you will be surprised to see the headline" Happy birthday Rishabh"..or "Happy birthday kanika..." There is a tradition to write the name of the child with birthday wishes on the case sheet on their birthday so every Doctor, Sister and staff wish them and brightens their day. You will find these kids singing, playing, laughing and enjoying every bit of their life left. I have seen kids bouncing back to their music and dance straight from their chemo bed. I wonder from where they get this enormous strength and energy. I haven't seen Dr Appaji taking any leave. He is single and solely dedicated to his profession,his patients are his family. We used to doze off in the post lunch classes but Dr Appaji never failed to teach us every aftrnoon. His powerpoint presentation are still alive in my mind. Such a dedicated man! Man of few words but man of enormous knowledge.He is the literal meaning of dedication and i'm sure any people knowing him in person will agree to it wholely. Such people are gem and rare to find in current era.

Whenever i think of the exceptional and extraordinary Doctors,the name of my brother Late Dr Vinay Wali always lingers in my heart. No doubt he was my prime inspiration to be in this field. He was sensitive, sensible, emotional and humanitarian doctor.He was the one who always helped others out of his way to treat and cure. I have seen him paying room rents of his batchmates so they can continue their study and would not be drop outs from the colleges due to lack of money. Many of his friends passed their exam on my brother's books. He was the first doctor of his generation who revolutionalised computer technology to explain the diseases to his patients. He used to show them the pictures related to their diseases on the screen and used to explain it in simplified language.He never worked for money but moreover treated freely poor and the needy patients. His doors were always open to all the needy and ailing people of all caste and creed.

I have seen him crying when his patient lost his battle against illness. I have seen him carrying old patient in his arms in emergency and saving life. I have seen him paying money from his pocket so that poor patients can go to higher centre for their treatment. I used to get pissed off with his calls with referring the patients to our tertiary hospital where i was studying Mbbs as it was my job to take his patients to respective wards and give him daily updates about their wellbeing. But i knew he was a Man of gold! I have seen him sharing his food with the hungry people sitting in the corridors of the hospital and even donating his own blood for his needy patients.He had a mass connect and was hugely popular among his peers and patients. He had a huge fan following, had best handwriting, excellent drawing skills,melodious voice. He was an expert musician and the tech savvy. He was a decade ahead in science and technology, was the best goal keeper of his football team,State level winner of science project and his theme of switching off the street lights at the onset of sun rays was hugely appreciated by whole India. He was the only person selected from the entire Maharashtra in the National cadet corp(NCC) and represented Maharashtra at National level.He was the first in the merit list in his 10th board exam and the winner of Best outgoing student award in school and colleges.He had put the stage on fire with his rocking performances in our social gatherings.He was no doubt a wonderful doctor but more than that a wonderful humanbeing for his patients. Whatsoever short life he lived he lived it king size! Some lives are destined to live for others! No doubt he was a real champion!!

People like Dr Appaji, Dr Vinay Wali,Dr Baba Amte, Dr Prakash Amte enlight us that there are doctors who work beyond the boundaries of time,money and notion of getting rich.They live simple life yet setting high examples for the people who know them and see them.Despite the negativity spread by the few sick and mean minded people by the paid media and politicians thirsty for the votes trying to tarnish images of Doctors and medical fraternity Doctors like Appaji sir,my brother, my Dad, Dr Amte and all other known and unknown doctors striving hard to save lives are like dhruva tara shining high in all the adversities and proving the worth to be in this noble profession. I have not seen any god till date but i worship him with all faith and hence the doctors like these are the Visible Gods for me. I'm proud of this white coat and jewel of stethoscope around my neck earned from my sweat and blood and i feel proud to dedicate my life to this noble profession of saving life.Today on the occasion of Doctors Day i salute all these real life heroes,all the doctors who are working relentlessly day and night in any nook and corner of the world to make difference in someone's life giving us will to proceed positively " Ruka jaana nahi tu kahi haar k; ki kaaton pe chalake mile hai saayien bahar ke" these lines are apt for these selfless creatures! Visible gods they are indeed..!!

* * *

CHAPTER 38

BABUMOSHAI ONE MORE TIME

"Ba Aadab, Ba Mulahija,hoshiyar.... Babumoshai padhar rahe hai....!!"Our canteen boy raju announced cheekily as he put the glasses of hot cups of tea in front of us at our busy opd tables.And then came flying white Gandhi topi of our harikaka,our opd attendant followed by he himself searching for his topi muttering bit furiously the "Demon is here".Wide smile got spread on all of our faces as we knew our Babu moshai has arrived. He needs no introduction.He is a very enthusiastic,fairly hyperactive guy Golu! He was fondly called as Golu because of his oversized & heavy weight body. But he used to take immense pleasure to call himself Babumoshai as he was very filmy who kept enacting various roles of famous characters from hit movies and kept us entertaining to the core.

Film Anand being his most favourite one. His visit to our hospital was funtime in our opd which we all Doctors enjoyed a lot. I was working in the Government Medical college after my post graduation and these were the kids from Karuna Bhavan,an orphanage for the children with AIDS.The children from this place used to come to us routinely for their all health aliments.

OPD sister called him.Tell me your name, have to write in our opd register she said in a plain tired voice." Iss Nachiz ko Golu bulate hai,Naam toh suna hi hoga" But aap mujhe pyar se Dholu bula sakte hai"...He said cheesily in his nautanki way and we all rolled laughing our hearts out. He was a 13-14 years old boy from Karuna Bhavan who used to visit us regularly. He was known asthamatic and seasonal variations used to often worsen his plight.

Salaam Madamji, mereku thoda sardi jaise lagri and halak mei kaise kaise kich toh hora he said in the typical hyderabadi slang as he knew I was Hyderabad Return. Ok...haibath haibat nakko karu, mai tumarko dawaiya likh deti hun, goli daal lo, sab khariyat hoga phir i too replied in my typical hyderabadi urdu style and the entire OPD bursted out in laughter.This boy always brought lots of energy and fun vibes to the surrounding. I prescribed him medications and he left again by throwing hari kakas white Gandhi topi in the air and saying phir miltun hari kaka tab tak Jai Jai Ram Krishna Hari and to the nurse he said madamji next time yaad rakhna,Golu naam toh suna hi hai na ab! And he walked away leaving behind his thunderous laughter.

Kahan se aati hai inme itni himmat? I thought to myself. Their life is dark and future is bleak.Their days are uncertain and hence they live today to the fullest as if there is no tomorrow. No parents, no trace of their relatives,they live as orphans.Kids like them in the orphanage are their siblings and caretakers of Karuna Bhavan their family.Their living depends on the people's charity.Some one's birthday and someone's death anniversary celebrations are their feast days.Some days they have very little to eat but still they share what they have in their plate.They take care of each others in their sickness and they literally coexist with each other.Really some relations are not Man made, but are truly God Made in every sense.

Children suffering from Aids are still tabood in our so called educated and civilised society. They are disowned and often left on their own fate. But still these kids live happily in their innocent world totally unaware of the gravity of their underlying health issues.They just know they have Aids but dont know it's long term complications and consequences. Keeping their CD4 count under check and taking medications under HAART regime is their daily routine.Their immune system is weak and they are often prone to each and every opportunistic infection. Don't know why God is so unkind and cruel to some kids.

I used to visit Karuna Bhavan to meet these kids for their health check up once in a while as a part of social service. Golu used to be their Gang leader arranging all the kids in a queue and bringing them for the check up and dictating everyone's complaint.He was everyone's Big B there!

"He is a very sensitive and kind madam, he shows as if he is very funny and carefree but he takes utmost care of every child here. If someone is sick he nurse them whole day-night and keeps praying with teary eyes"..Vidhya Tai the caretaker of Karuna Bhavan was telling me about Golu. I couldn't miss her moist eyes. Humanity still exist in this materialistic world I said to her looking into her deep eyes.

A few days later as I was busy winding up my opd there he came...Golu but this time looking sick and breathless.He came walking with vidhyatai and two of his inmates holding his hands.Hari kaka,tumhari topi salamat hai aaj, yeh log pakad k rakhe hai na haath he tried smiling faintly. Acute exacerbation of Asthma i said.Immediately we admitted him in the ICU and started oxygen therapy, antibiotics and nebulization with close monitoring of his vitals.Few days down the lane he was feeling much better but still required minimal oxygen and hence we shifted him to the ward. Everyday his friends used to visit him and they used to have a gala time together.They used to sing, joke and dance.Golu used to go to every patient enquiring about their health and make them laugh with his stupid entertaining jokes. He used to get daily hot pipping fresh food from his orphanage but he never failed to share his meals with his friends who were other patients in his ward.Isse kehte hai Daryadili !! Their loud talks used to disturb the santity of the entire ward still people loved his intelligent talks and every night was Golu's entertainment programme with his mimicry of popular actors.His dialouges from salman khan's Dabhang movie,his mimicry of shahrukh khan used to make nights there a laugh riot! Head Nurse used to scold him,this is hospital not your theatrical stage,Go and sleep now and let others sleep too."kaiku pukare mummy, logon ko hasaye toh woh jaldi theek hote" he used to enlighten her. And as she goes out for dinner,the ward used to turn into a dancing floor with all the kids dancing on zingat tunes.Golu was seen holding his oxygen pipe in nose and dancing whole heartedly.Don't stress yourself Golu, you will feel breathless, take rest..ward nurses used to warn him.I'm fine now, "Zindagi Ek baar hi milti hai senorita, khul k jeeni chahiye, kya pata kal ho na ho"!He used to tell them in a filmy way. So notorious and filmy he is..ward sisters used to say fondly.

I want to go home Vidyatai idhar ka show time hogaya mera,next day he was telling painfully.I could sense he was missing his home, his friends and playmates.We discharged him telling to take rest and to take utmost precautions.

A week later at night my phone rang. "Madam...Vidyatai here, Golu's condition has worsened for bad.He is very breathless we are getting him to the hospital now"she said hurriedly. I rushed to the emergency ward racing my car. I could see Golu lying very weak and with severe breathing difficulty,Spo2 in 80's.They got me directly here in ER so that I won't fly hari kaka's topi and won't trouble your OPD nurse.This is cheating na madamji, he tried to joke and smile but could hardly talk and hardly breath.

We started him on the respiratory support, iv fluids, antibiotics and other supportive treatment.His chest xray showed pneumocystitis Carinii pneumonia. Deadly pneumonia in the patients with Aids.His CD4 counts have dropped very low. I knew it was a very critical condition and chances of his recovery was very very less.

Whole night I waited in ICU applying my whole knowledge to save this brave Ninja.But sometimes body power falls low and even greatest warrior throw his armours down.I could see him sinking.We will ventilate him I told worriedly to sobbing Vidhya Tai.Nahi Madam Ji " Zindagi badi honi chahiye, Lambi nahi, hum toh sab iss rangmanch k katputali hai, jiska role khatam usko exit lena chahiye.Mera life picture ab khatam hogaya hai, exit lene ka waqt hai.Mujhe aap sab k saath haste bolte hi jaana hai"he spoke feebly.His oxygen levels started dropping to the critical level, heart rate started falling.He could see all his friends cum family members from Karuna Bhavan standing near the glass wall and crying,trying to have a glimpse of him.He raised his hand for final good bye and breathed his last.

I have saved hundreds of lives in my career yet have seen many deaths. But this death shattered me to the core.Doctors are trained to be empathetic but sometimes humanity overpowers our profession.Heart rules our head. Don't know if Death made his life easier but his absence will create a big vaccum in the hearts of many whom he nurtured and cared.Today my eyes were flowing along with hues n cries of his friends and family from Karuna Bhavan. Even Hari kaka cried who will fly my topi now Golu? The blockbuster Golu's show was off air from our OPD permanently now. But the character of Golu was permanently etched in everyone's memory whom he met and he touched all the lives.His partying in wards along with his mates and singing chalte chalte mere yeh geet yaad rakhna, kabhi alvida na kehna, kabhi alvida na kehna kept repeating and rewinding in front of my eyes! Kabhi tumhe Alvida nahi bol sakte Dost, tum toh har ek k Dil mei basne wale superstar ho. Bhale hi tum zindagi se haare, but tumne toh kaha tha,

"Haar kar jitne wale ko hi Bazigar kehte hai"! Yes you lived by your saying "zindagi badi honi chahiye babumoshai lambi nahi"!You lived your life like a king and ruled all the hearts.Jaha bhi ho bas khush raho. I turned around with my whirling thoughts and started walking wiping my tears. It seemed like the world had come to the halt and time machine has frozen.Everything in front of my eyes was dark and deep.Really some people brings light to our lives.And Golu you were the shining candle who melted yourself making others life brighter! You were and will remain the most loved superstar forever alive in all our hearts !!!

* * *

CHAPTER 39

WHEN I MET MY VITTHU-MAULI

I just love road trips and we keep doing random ones frequently.Our car speeds on the newly built 6 lane highway on the Pandharpur Kolhapur road.We were just returning from Pandharpur,Tuljapur Darshan.Clouds were clear, it was a pleasant evening.Sun was ready to set, cool breeze gave us refreshing feeling.The Sky was coloured with red,maroon,golden,mauve,the golden rays making the sky more colourful and bright.Road was clean,the highway was beautified with green trees standing tall on the sides and waving us with their green leaves.Intermittent cool showers of rain made the atmosphere more serene.What a bliss...real it was! It was the month of Ashaad the holy month of hindu calender moresoever striking month in maharashtra where lakhs of devotees flock eagerly and walks miles and miles towards Pandharpur to meet their Lord Vitthal desperately.

I always loved the bond between the Lord Vitthal and his devotees.It's a bond of the mother and child.His devotees walks from every nook and corner of Maharashtra.They are old,they are poor,bent in their spine yet they have this child like energy which keeps them walking through the dawn and dusk, through the dust and rain,dancing,singing merged in the devotion of Lord Vitthu Mauli with the eagerness of a child to meet his mother and when they meet their Mother- Mauli vitthal it's just so pure and divine. It's a very emotional and spectacular view where lakhs of devotees put their forehead and wet His feet with their tears of love and joy.This is the most purest abhishek any Lord can ever have! This union of the Lord and his devotees is more pure and holy than any sangam of holy river.

Vitthal is the mother of poor and needy who lives under the sky, works barefootedly in the farms and mud, the people whose belief in their mauli is unshaken.Lord works with them in their farms and eat the roti and curry from their hardworking hands.This Aashadi vaari as famously called as Dindi in maharashtra is a spectacular view to watch and moresoever the moments to cherish for life.

As we travelled across the highway we could see many many groups of vaarkaris (vitthal Bhakts) wearing white clothes,tulsi mala around their neck, playing taal- mrudang in their hands, singing Abhang(famous songs of lord vitthal) and traversing their path with saffron flags in their hands.We were taken aback with their energy, stamina in this age.This Vaarkari Sampraday running their legacy for hundreds of years now is the pride of every Maharashtrian and I deeply believe that the Guiness book of World record should take a note of this greatly organised largest peaceful march involving lakhs of people showcasing the rich cultural heritage of our country.But these people in this vaari are above all these riches, awards and records.They are simple souls who are just embarked in the devotion and Bhakti of their Mauli.Their whole world revolves around their kanada Vitthal.And their Lord too is waiting from the decades to decades eagerly to meet his children.Their bond is just straight from heart, it cannot be told,it cannot be sold, it cannot be measured but is only treasured by the TRUE Vitthal Bhakts!!

Looking at these vaarkari i suddenly went into the flash back.It was a decade ago where during the similar season of Aashad Vaari a couple brought their two kids to our hospital.It was hot sunny afternoon and these couple carried their children in their arms.There is this emergency madam, i think you should see them quickly. My senior nurse opened the door and intrupted me.I knew it was a real emergency as she otherwise won't intrupt me when i'm seeing some patient. I handed over the prescription to my patient in my OPD and rushed to the Emergency. When they alert me of any emergency I have this peculiar picture in mind, One serious patient lying on the bed, mob of attenders surrounding the bed trying to create rukus and our nursing staff trying to squeeze their way through this crowd to give the patient first aid.

With worried look i entered the ER but to my surprise, there was no mob,no noise, no tensed air.I thought for a while did she really informed me about the emergency? I looked around when our senior sister came out of the cubicle, this way mam, she guided me. I entered the cubicle to find out two young children aged 7 years and 5 years lying on the beds nearby. They looked dehydrated. Their parents were simple village clad people. Father was dressed in white payjama and cotton shirt and wore white gandhi topi on his head.Mother was wrapped in a simple cotton green saree. Both had tulsi mala around the neck and black tilak on their forehead hallmark of Vitthal Bhakts.They stood there in a corner calm and composedly joining their hands. In no time I knew they were Vaarkaris going for Aashad Vaari to the Pandharpur. They are vomiting frequently, not eating or drinking anything since yesterday so have to get them here they told in a soft voice.

I turned to examine them and i was shocked to find out both

their children were special child with full blown Cerebral palsy,Mental retardation and contractures. They were affected with hot scorching sun outside and were dehydrated. I immediately started them on iv fluids,ORS as they tolerated and other supportive measures.After an hour or so their vitals normalised and hydration got better.

I took the parents to my cabin.Made them sit in a cool place.Offered them water and ordered some snacks and fruits for them. From where are you?and how you are travelling to Pandharpur with these children i asked them curiously. They were from nearby village on Telangana- Maharashtra border. Ardent followers of Lord vitthal who travel to Pandharpur every year with these children of their's with special needs. Every year we carry them on our shoulders or in our arms.They tolerated odd weathers and sun all these years. But this year sun is too hot and they couldn't eat anything and got dehydrated they told innocently. Snacks arrived which they polietly denied but i forcefully made them to eat fruits and to have some cool buttermilk. They looked little better now.Don't you feel sad having these babies with special needs? People get depressed and agitated having one child like this and you are having two. Both bed ridden,how do you handle them? I wanted to know.

Madam, We got married in close relation and have this genetic problem running in our families. Doctor said our all kids might face similar problems.They simply smiled looking at the sky but we know that "they are our Pandurang(vitthal). He has gifted these two innocent souls to us." These kids dont know who are they, they dont understand what they are suffering. They are as pure and innocent like our Vitthu Mauli. They smile when we pick them and care for them. They are happy when we feed them. They love us to the core and have imparted us the blessing of parenthood.We feel specially chosen as their parents by our Lord to take care of them.To serve them we feel we are serving our Lord. They are not burden to us madam but God has given us this chance to serve Him through these two kids.And we will care for them till our last breath they told firmly.

They may not be able to do things on their own. But their face shines with happiness when we sing abhang, they dance waving their hands when we hail vitthal vitthal jai hari vitthal.They gave us the opportunity to be the parents and we are indebted to them for this they told with moist eyes.How long we need to be here madam? we need to reach Pandharpur before Ekadashi he informed me.I told them not to worry as they were getting better. Its just dehydration due to severe heat.They will be alright soon and vitthal is there with us right? i said positively. They nodded with a smile. Till evening both of them got better. Both parents were sitting next to them caring whole heartedly wiping their faces and talking to them.My heart melted to see them.

We are arranging food for you Dada tonight i informed him. No madam, really we can't take this we dont have much money to pay you for your treatment, can't afford paying for this food again they refused politely.Dada you have given me opportunity to serve Lord Vitthal today.You people are true hardcore Vitthal Bhakts and serving you is like serving God so let me do this honour.And haa, I know your self respect so I won't give you anything for free neither my treatment nor the food.You have to repay me for both i told him bit sternly. How can we repay you madam? his wife asked in shivering tone. I patted her softly and said vaarkaris are here, Dindi is going on and how come my place will go without bhajan. You have to sing abhang and we will have small Bhajan gathering here tonight i told them my wish. They were more than happy to know that they won't go missing on their prayers tonight.

Our enthusiastic staff arranged mattresses in the front hall. We arranged Vitthal- Rukmini photo on the table, did puja.We invited some Vitthal Bhakts from our local temple and they came happily with taal,mridunga,veena and what happened after that was the history. It was a fully devotional night with melodious Abhang,vitthal bhajans.The sound waves of this melodious music went in the every nook and corner of our hospital making it more pious.Every place was energised. Patients felt some divine energy chanellising them. Everyone had a sense of well being.The whole atmosphere turned so positive and divine.The power of music as a therapy to heal i was experiencing it live today.Even the two kids with special needs participated in the Abhang waving their hands.Our staff did zimma,fugadi and ringan dance along with these Vaarkaris.Vitthal gajar made the night so pure and aesthetic.This was one night to remember. People felt so happy and everyone had the hearty hot meals together. Everyone including me had a very deep and peaceful sleep after eons of years.

Next day i got up early, got ready instantly and went to the hospital by 7am. The children looked bright and hydrated. Their faces looked more cheerful now and they gave me familiar smile as they have seen me with them last night.They all looked so fresh in their clean white clothes.Children were also ready with naam on their forehead and black tika amidst the white chandan naam.We served them freshly made breakfast and tea.Till then our ambulance driver arrived.We gifted them fruit baskets and all sat in ambulance and waved our staff. I said i will too accompany you till you meet your vaarkari friends on the way. We had traced them and they weren't too far.They were halting in a nearby village almost 25 kms from our place. We drove quickly and dropped them in their group. All their team mates were so happy to meet these people. All women and men older in age hugged these two little kids.The happiness to see them healthy and joining back the troupe was clearly seen flowing on their faces.First time I could see these children with special needs treated so warmly and with so much love. Other healthy men carried them on their shoulders."Chala Mauli we will leave now" said the father.You met us like our God and treated our kids so affectionately they said in a teary voice."No no Dada because of you I got an opportunity to serve Vithoba from my place itself.I can't go to vaari and can't walk to pandharpur like you all. So maybe God only came to meet me in your form" i was bit emotional by now. All started walking dived in devotion of their Great Lord.The sound of taal ,mrudang and Abhang filled up the sky. Two special children were sitting on the shoulders of these vaarkari men.Crowd slowly went far and far.I could see the images of Vitthal and Rukmini sitting on the shoulders of those two men and guiding them to the way of pandharpur."Paule Chalati Pandharichi Waat"...I could hear this famous marathi song in the background.Finally Vitthu mauli met his children...And I could see my vitthal today in them!

* * *

CHAPTER 40
HUMAN PYRAMID

Life is a mixed bag of emotions.All emotions...happy,sad, joy,anger,envy and surprise.In the school we were always taught that "Man is a social animal and life makes all sense with the people around".We cross each other's path for a reason.Each and every person we meet are of different personalities,different nature and different thought process and that's what makes Life more interesting!! Imagine a life without human interactions,no one to share and no one to care,how difficult it sounds.Yeah how much ever money we make,earning our own people who will be there with us in every thick and thin of our life is the greatest asset.Truly rich is a person who earns more people than money and in that sense i find my parents to be the luckiest.

My Dad is the first doctor in our entire family.Genius by birth and hardworking by nature he has mastered the skill of clinical practice so well that he is famous among his peers and the society for his best treatment.Poor people's doctor is what he is fondly called as.After completion of his internship,post MBBS he was posted in a far off hilly area in the Satara district of Maharashtra as a Government Doctor and he inaugurated the first PHC there at Jawale.People there were so glad to have the Medical facility and a good qualified Doctor now at their bay. In a very short span he was very popular and hundreds of people from all the neighbouring villages,towns and district started visiting him and his treatment story spread too far.Very poor,needy,vulnerable people used to flock daily and my father was examining them and treating them whole day and night.My mother bought up in a very developed area and cosmopolitan culture felt like she was missing on some deserted island staying there but for my father's passion she too got adjusted soon.

Devoid of the basic facilities of road, electricity and transport it was very difficult for the people to reach PHC in time.They used to carry sick people in cloth zholi walking miles away on the thorns and stones to reach my father and with my Dad's Midas touch they used to feel better instantly.As a token of appreciation and gratitude they used to get basket full of green leafy vegetables, fruits, grains and millets,coconuts,groundnuts and kharwas for us to eat.Small babies were wrapped in a warm saree and they used to bring them in a small basket keeping on their head walking and crossing the river midway with the only hope for their near and dear ones in form of my father and he lived upto their expectations always.

After serving them for 3 years my father came back to my native and started his own clinical practice in my hometown but our bond with the people of that village never dimmed.From 300 kms they kept on visiting my dad for their aliments.Once in our primary school days when we had been on a trip,on our return we halted back to meet those villagers.In one of our known people's house we loved a golden kitten with furry tail.It was royal and elegant and we developed instant liking towards it.But as we were traveling far we couldn't get him along with us.But somewhere deep in our hearts we weren't able to forget that Golden furry ball.And to our surprise after few days that owner got that kitten to us putting it into small basket and that baby cat travelled in a public bus to reach us.Such was the love,affection and loyalty of those people towards their very first Doctor who laid the foundation of Medical facilities in their remote village.Being kids we used to sometimes sit at our clinic's reception and see varities of patients of different age groups,caste,creed and religion coming to us for their treatment.Their dresses,language and living style was very different from each other but they were all same at their hearts.Their emotions were equal and mainly they all had immense faith and respect for my father.He treated many poor patients for free and for most of our relatives he helped in their crisis for education and building their careers but never made a hype out of it.He always believes less is more and simple living and high thinking is his mantra.

I still remember two young burkha clad Muslim girls visiting our clinic regularly.We used to chat with them and they used to sing for us"Chasma utaro phir dekho yaaro yeh duniya badi rangeen hai..chasme badhur" was their favourite song and we remembered them as song wale ladkiya.The poor farm workers from small and deep villages of Karnataka used to come during harvesting season in and around our town to cut sugarcane and transport them to sugar factories.Staying in the cold environment of the farms they used to often get cold, fever,allergies and pneumonia.These people used to come to my Dad for treatment but we never know till date how they used to come to know about my father only when many other options were available in my town."Garibon ka Wali Doctor" they call him fondly! And my father treats everyone equal without seeing their caste, creed, religion or financial status.

We have this Irani muslim clan at my place.Our municipality has donated them some lands where they have made their permanent habitat.Their small huts are fully loaded with every amenities and facilities.They have small TV, transistor, bed,fan everything in that small place.They generally are carefree people who live for today and won't bother about tomorrow.They sell cooling glasses, gents belts,perfumes and some small items roadside but they never interfere with the locals here.They have matriarchy system in their tribe and one old lady in late 60's is their head boss.Anyone sick and ailing she accompany them to our clinic.We used to be initially very scared looking at them but my father told they are good people, they don't steal or rob or do any kind of ruckus.They earn their own bread and butter and live happily within their tribe.They are "Harfan Maulas" my Dad used to say and they never missed to pay my Dad's meager fee.

Still i remember after our SSLC board exams we had been to Chinchali Mayyaka temple somewhere in Karnataka.They had annual fair (jatra) there of the Goddess who is very famous and thought to be very powerful.After darshan we were walking down the streets looking at colourful toys and jwellery shops arranged in a row beautifully flaunting their colourful items.We heard some one calling us.She was a middle aged lady running her sugarcane juice shop in that jatra.We didn't knew them but she was a regular patient of my Dad and she saw and recognised my father and invited us all to her shop and offered us chilled sweet sugarcane juice free of cost.Really these poor people have rich hearts....i always believe.

Some patients become so familiar that we start feeling them like a part of our family. Deluxe tailor who runs his tailoring shop in our lane sends us litres of sheer kurma every Ramadan and Doni family who gets us chonge (Coconut poli) at Muharram are the Muslims who are age old patients of my Dad. One lady from neighbouring village used to consult my father for her health issues regularly.Her entire family used to come to us.Everytime she used to visit she used to carry fresh vegetables from her farm and my grandmother used to serve her hot tea and then both used to chat for long times.There was no rich and poor, there was no educated and uneducated difference but it was only the sharing,hearing and caring.This was the bonding of pure souls. No business,no gains but only affection and that's why these kinds of bonds were stronger and lasted for eons together!

The road construction workers, the gold dust collection people who collect dust outside the jewellery shop and separate small minute gold and silver particles, Municipality sweeper Sanju who clean our roads daily all visit my Dad for their aliments and he treats them with care and dignity.

In our childhood every Sunday after weekly bazaar we used to see a very old lady collecting grains fallen on the ground and used to seperate good vegetables from the heaps thrown on the road at the end of market hours.She didn't had any money to buy her daily essentials but she had this hope that if she falls sick my father will treat her for meager amount and she will get back to her work the very next day with full energy. Really he has this Midas touch! We feel proud and happy to see so many poor unaffording people getting perfectly alright with my fathers treatment and going home happily.He is a man of principles and his healing touch has brightened lives of so many!!

Looking at all these people who regularly visit us i feel they all are the part of Human Pyramid.Different people of different strata,different languages, different cultural backgrounds but together they form a symbol of humanity, brotherhood and mankind.They always taught us that together we stand stronger.We are really blessed to see these all kind of people and their lives so closely. My parents taught us with their own behaviour to treat everyone equal and with due respect.There is no rich, no poor, no small or big in our house but everyone is human.My Grandmother always said we need all kinds of people around us as each and every person has some unique qualities and every one is important in one or other way.That's the reason we are always grounded and connected to our roots.After all to reach the pinnacle of success we need the foundation of trust and solidarity and this Human Pyramid serves it all!! These people around us help us to climb to the top of this Human Pyramid with ease and elan.These all small and big people of various caste,creed and religion makes a huge human pyramid who binds us together and form the firm base of our lives. And that's why I feel we are more richer and royal in our hearts!!

* * *

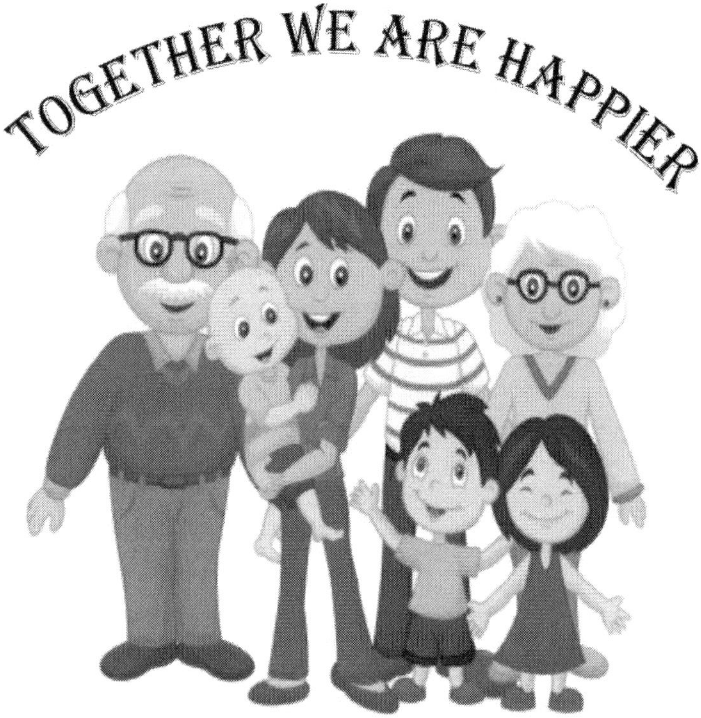
TOGETHER WE ARE HAPPIER

Made in United States
Orlando, FL
05 November 2026

90230145R00138